READING DISABILITIES

AF788065

NEUROPSYCHOLOGY AND COGNITION

VOLUME 4

Series Editor:

R. Malatesha Joshi, *Oklahoma State University, U.S.A.*

Advisory Board:

Alfonso Caramazza, *The Johns Hopkins University, U.S.A.*

George Hynd, *University of Georgia, U.S.A.*

C.K. Leong, *The University of Victoria, Canada*

John Marshall, *University of Oxford, U.K.*

Gabriele Miceli, *Università Cattolica Del Sacro Cuore, Italy*

Loraine Obler, *City University of New York, U.S.A.*

Sandra Witelson, *McMaster University, Canada*

The purpose of the Neuropsychology and Cognition series is to bring out volumes that promote understanding in topics relating brain and behavior. It is intended for use by both clinicians and research scientists in the fields of neuropsychology, cognitive psychology, psycholinguistics, speech and hearing, as well as education. Examples of topics to be covered in the series would relate to memory, language acquisition and breakdown, reading, attention, developing and aging brain. By addressing the theoretical, empirical, and applied aspects of brain-behavior relationships, this series will try to present the information in the fields of neuropsychology and cognition in a coherent manner.

The titles published in this series are listed at the end of this volume.

Reading Disabilities

Genetic and Neurological Influences

Edited by
BRUCE F. PENNINGTON
University of Denver, U.S.A.

Reprinted from *Reading and Writing*, Volume 3, Nos. 3-4 (1991)

SPRINGER-SCIENCE+BUSINESS MEDIA, B.V

ISBN 978-94-010-5081-4 ISBN 978-94-011-2450-8 (eBook)
DOI 10.1007/978-94-011-2450-8

All Rights Reserved
© 1991 Springer Science+Business Media Dordrecht
Originally published by Kluwer Academic Publishers in 1991
Softcover reprint of the hardcover 1st edition 1991
No part of the material protected by this copyright notice may be reproduced or utilized in any form or by any means, electronic or mechanical, including photocopying, recording or by any information storage and retrieval system, without written permission from the copyright owner.

(on acid-free paper)

Contents

PART THREE: Discussion

Overview

Genetic and Neurological Influences on Reading Disability: An Overview

BRUCE F. PENNINGTON

University of Denver, U.S.A.

ORIGINS

This special issue grew out of the XVI International Rodin Remediation Scientific Conference held in Boulder, Colorado in September, 1990 which was devoted to the topic of genetic and neurological influences on dyslexia, or reading disability (RD). This conference would not have been possible without the vision and generosity of Per Udden and the Rodin Remediation Foundation, who have been unique catalysts in fostering an interdisciplinary understanding of dyslexia or RD.

This conference was special both scientifically and personally. Scientifically, this was the first time that most of the world's experts on the genetics and neurology of RD all gathered at the same meeting, although subsets of these research communities have met at previous meetings. Moreover, because of recent advances in both fields, the outlines of a complete neuroscientific understanding of this prevalent, complex behavioral disorder was finally within our grasp; the proof of this perhaps bold assertion is contained in the papers that follow. The 1990s had been dubbed "The Decade of the Brain" and this meeting was one of several fitting inaugurals of this decade.

Personally, this was a poignant occasion because one of the world's pioneers in reading research, Isabelle Liberman, had died unexpectedly a few months before. The conference included a tribute to her. Her close collaborators, Don Shankweiler and Susan Brady, both delivered moving reminiscences about her life and work. Alvin Liberman, her husband and fellow scientist, was there to be part of that tribute. As Isabelle certainly would have wished, he also attended the conference and served as a stimulating, *ad hoc* discussant, presenting the views on reading that Isabelle, he and other co-workers have so impressively developed. He also contributed a formal discussion to this volume.

Sadly, another loss followed the conference. Karen Gross-Glenn, a cognitive scientist working on visual and neuroanatomical differences in RD in collaboration with Herbert Lubs, died in November, 1990. She was one of the presenters at the conference, and will be sorely missed.

Reading and Writing: An Interdisciplinary Journal 3: 191–201, 1991.
© 1991 *Kluwer Academic Publishers.*

INTRODUCTION TO THE ISSUE: CONVERGENCES AND DIVERGENCES

I have tried to organize the papers in this volume to emphasize both convergences and divergences in our emerging understanding of the neuroscience of RD, and I will sketch out my sense of these here. Hopefully, this introduction will make the volume more accessible to readers not versed in the technical complexities of behavior genetics and neuroimaging.

Despite these complexities, the overall significance of the genetic results presented here are straightforward: RD runs in families (familiality); this familiarlity is partly due to genetic influence (heritability); these heritable influences act more on the phonological than the orthographic aspect of word recognition (differential heritability), both in RD and normal subjects; and we are beginning to locate some of the genes that may be influencing RD (gene locations).

While these genes ultimately influence RD, it would be misleading to say there are genes specifically for either normal or abnormal reading ability, since reading *per se* was never subject to natural selection in evolution. Instead, spoken language and other behavioral skills that proved adaptive were selected for in human evolution. Only behavioral variations that were genetically based could be selected and maintained by natural selection, so human, species-typical cognitive characteristics, such as spoken language, must have a genetic and therefore physical basis, most likely in the brain. It could be that variations *within* our species in spoken language facility and other cognitive skills are entirely environmental, in contrast to the clear genetic basis for differences in these skills *between* species. However, it is quite plausible that there would be genetically-based, within-species variation, especially for recently evolved skills such as spoken language. Variations in some of these spoken language and possibly other cognitive skills could in turn have effects on reading skill; hence there would, indirectly, be genetic influences on reading skill. As the reader will see, there is both convergence and controversy about the precise nature of the cognitive and neurological phenotype that is genetically influenced in RD.

Before proceeding further, it is important to address another frequent but mistaken inference about the implications of genetic influence on RD, this time in the domain of treatment. Genetic influence on a disorder is a separate issue from whether or how the disorder can be treated. Many practitioners resist genetic interpretations because they fear they necessarily imply either untreatability or a biological (e.g., drug) treatment. But that is hardly the case. Some genetic disorders (e.g., phenylketonuria) are readily treatable, whereas some environmentally caused disorders (e.g., some effects of parental maltreatment) are not. Moreover, despite genetic influence on RD, the most efficacious available treatment is still behavioral (see Clark, 1988).

Returning to our main theme, the genetic influences on RD have implications for neuroimaging studies of RD. As indicated above, genetic influence on RD implies there is a physical basis for the trait, most likely in the brain and most likely in a specific part of the brain. Thus it makes sense to look for the neurological phenotype in RD (as well as in other genetically influenced behavior disorders). Obviously environmental influences also affect the physical structure of the brain, (unless one is a dualist), but likely in a different way than genetic ones. For instance, cultural influences on literacy would affect synapse strengths and dendritic branching, which are parameters of brain structure associated with learning (Greenough, Black and Wallace, 1987). If the genetic effects act early in development (as they must in an early appearing developmental disorder like RD), then the parameters of brain structure affected would be ones such as neuronal number, neuronal migration and axonal connectivity, which are determined with few exceptions before birth.

Neuroimaging is a newer specialty than behavior genetics, and there are naturally more technical issues and complexities. Nonetheless, the papers in this volume indicate an encouraging degree of convergence on what the neurological phenotype in RD may be. Several independent studies have found alterations in the size and symmetry of the planum temporale, a posterior structure in the neocortex which contributes to the processing of phonology in speech. The planum thus makes theoretical sense as being *part* of the neurological phenotype in RD. There are other reasons discussed below why it is unlikely to be the necessary and sufficient neurological phenotype in RD.

So much for the "big picture," which at this point is very exciting — so exciting that we may be tempted to gloss over discrepancies and gaps in our knowledge. What I will do next is introduce each paper in each section in turn, highlighting both its relation to others and the empirical and theoretical issues that it raises.

Genetics

These papers are arranged in order of the series of linked questions we can ask of a behavioral phenotype like RD. First, is it familial? The paper by Gilger, Pennington, and DeFries provides clear evidence of familiality from four samples, replicating earlier results from several studies. Although risk to first degree relatives varies understandably with the definition of RD and how the sample was ascertained, this familial risk is clearly significant and substantial in all samples studied. As every clinician knows, many RD children have RD parents. So the fact of familiality in RD is a well-established one. The next question is whether this familiality is due to genetic or environmental factors, or both.

If entirely environmental, we would expect the preschool literacy environment to be systematically different in RD vs. non-RD families. The second paper by Scarborough, which provides additional evidence for the familiality of RD, shows this is *not* the case. Differences in the pre-school literacy environment between RD and non-RD families appear to be mainly specific to the children *within* RD families who later become RD. There are not differences found for all children in RD families, at least in this middle class sample. In other words, there is not evidence in this study for what a behavioral geneticist would call common family environment effects — aspects of the pre-school literacy environment that affect all children in a family equally, although such effects very likely operate in some subcultures in our society. Instead there is evidence of what a behavior geneticist would call specific environmental effects — aspects of the environment which differ among children in the same family. In Scarborough's study, these specific environment effects appear to be child-driven, in part; the future RD children were less interested in literacy experiences at an early age. These child-driven, specific environmental differences could be thought of as examples of what a behavior geneticist would call reactive, and even active, genetic-environmental correlation (Scarr and McCartney, 1983). Genes and environment do not necessarily act independently. Instead, it makes sense to suppose that a child's genotype affects how the environment reacts to the child and what kind of environmental "niche" the child builds for herself. So pre-RD children appear to be creating an environmental niche that is less based on literacy experiences, even at an early age! Scarborough's paper is also important because it demonstrates for the first time that there is an early linguistic phenotype in RD. Syntax as well as phonology appear to be part of the early linguistic phenotype in RD, broadening our notions of how language development is affected in RD.

Scarborough's paper also has implications for the neurological phenotype in RD. It is theoretically possible, but unlikely, that the genes affecting RD affect a late brain developmental event, such as the myelination of the corpus callosum. If that were true, there might be *no* behavioral phenotype until that brain milestone was reached. Instead, Scarborough's data demonstrate there is a behavioral phenotype detectable as early as 30 months. Consequently, the changes in brain development must be earlier still.

To really know if the familiality of RD is in part genetic, we need results from methodologies that unconfound genetic and environmental influences. The methodology used to address this issue in RD has been the twin method; the two best twin studies of RD yet reported are both represented here, the Boulder and London studies. There are three papers from these two studies — the paper by Olson, Gillis, Rack, DeFries, and Fulker from the Boulder study, the paper by Stevenson from the London study, and a transatlantic collaboration found in the third paper by DeFries, Stevenson, Gillis, and Wadsworth. The consistency in results across the two studies is fairly striking. In both studies, deficits in phonological coding in RD are significantly more heritable than deficits in orthographic coding, and deficits in spelling are significantly and similarly heritable in both samples. The results of these twin studies provide the clearest evidence we have so far that RD is in part heritable. Moreover, the finding that deficits in specific components of the reading process are differentially heritable fits very nicely with results from the cognitive analysis of normal and abnormal reading. Deficits in the phonological coding of written language and the phonemic analysis of spoken language appear to be at the core of RD, and these deficits appear to be substantially heritable. In terms of divergences, there is a minor one. The Boulder sample has consistently found a heritable deficit in both real word reading and spelling scores in RD, whereas the London sample only finds this for spelling. These papers discuss possible reasons for this discrepancy, including differences in measures and age range of the samples.

The next genetic question concerns the mode of transmission, about which twin studies are ordinarily mute. A recent paper by our group (Pennington, Gilger, Pauls, Smith, Smith, and DeFries, in press), parts of which were presented at the Rodin meeting in Boulder, found evidence for major gene transmission (either additive or dominant) in a large proportion of RD families. This study examined four large samples of RD families ascertained through 204 RD probands ($N = 1686$ individuals). Thus, the genetic influences in RD may not be just classically polygenic, with hundreds (or thousands) of genes each contributing a small equal and additive effect. Instead, there may be a small set of genes of major effect which (indirectly) affect reading skill, in addition to a multitude of multifactors (including polygenes). Interestingly, this study also found a sex difference in penetrance of the putative major gene, with males being more penetrant. Attempting to eliminate this sex difference by setting the expected sex ratio to unity worsened the fit of the model to the data, so the obtained sex difference in penetrance is not just an artifact. Instead, in these samples of RD families, a slight excess of male dyslexics among adults appears to be a real phenomenon. If the childhood sex ratio is truly equal (Shaywitz, Shaywitz, Fletcher, and Escobar, 1990), then the adult sex difference could be produced by a sex difference in compensation (Lefly and Pennington, in press).

If there are genes of major effect, the next logical question is what is their location? This question cannot be addressed by the methodologies considered so far. Instead, linkage methods are needed which look for the cosegregation across generations of RD and a specific genetic marker(s).

The papers by Smith, Kimberling, and Pennington and Fulker, Cardon, DeFries, Kimberling, Pennington, and Smith both employ somewhat different forms of sibling pair linkage analysis to look for such cosegregation in the same data set. These data are from sibling pairs in extended families with three generation transmission of RD, previously studied for linkage using the traditional LOD score approach. Both studies found significant linkage of RD with chromosome 15 markers, a result which replicates our original result (Smith, Kimberling, Pennington, and Lubs, 1983). As Smith et al.'s paper points out, genetic heterogeneity has bedeviled traditional LOD score linkage analyses of RD (and other complex behavioral disorders). Because the sibling pair method is more flexible, it is less disrupted by genetic heterogeneity. Fulker et al.'s paper demonstrates that a multivariate regression approach to sibling pair linkage data in selected samples is very powerful indeed, with the power increasing with the degree of selection. Thus, this approach appears to be a useful way to screen the genome for loci affecting RD, as well as other behavioral traits.

Despite all these convergences, however, we still do not know in a definitive way if there is a major gene on chromosome 15 that is sufficient to cause RD. What we are detecting may not be a major gene, instead just a polygene, or it may not be there at all. The 15 results need to be confirmed in separate samples and in separate labs. The preliminary findings on chromosome 6 likewise need to be confirmed in other labs.

The last paper by Bender, Linden, and Robinson in this section provides definitive evidence that RD is genetically heterogeneous. One cause of RD is the sex chromosome anomaly 47, XXY. Because this anomaly is both non-familial and far too rare, it cannot account for the familiality or heritability of RD found in the other papers. Therefore, there must be at least two different genetic effects on RD, 47, XXY being one. (There are of course very likely more than two genetic effects on RD.)

Neurology and Neuropsychology

There are six papers in this section; the first four are concerned with direct measures of brain structure and function in relation to developmental differences in reading and language skill, and the last two are neuropsychological studies of RD, which have an indirect relation to brain structure and function.

As noted earlier, there is now converging evidence for a distinctive neurological phenotype in RD, which includes alterations in planum temporale symmetry, as well as other brain structure. The planum in the left hemisphere is part of Wernicke's area; the usual pattern of left greater than right planum asymmetry is thought to be a structural specialization that underlies the functional lateralization of certain language skills, especially phonological and syntactic ones, to the left hemisphere. Consequently, the finding by Galaburda and colleagues (Galaburda and Kemper, 1979; Galaburda, Sherman, Rosen, Aboitiz, and Geschwind, 1985) that there was an absence of planum asymmetry in dyslexic brains examined post mortem was of great theoretical interest. Only recently has it become possible to examine the planum *in vivo* using magnetic resonance imaging (MRI). Two independent studies using MRI (Hynd, Semrud-Clikeman, Lorys, Novey, and Eliopulos, 1990; Larsen, Hoien, Lundberg, and Odegaard, 1990) have found alterations in planum symmetry in living dyslexics. In the Hynd et al. study, there was a reversal of the usual L > R asymmetry, whereas in the Larsen et al. study there was a significant increase in symmetrical plana in the dyslexics, particularly those with phonological deficits. So the autopsy findings have generally been replicated using *in vivo* techniques.

The first four papers presented here carry this promising work forward partly by focusing on methodological issues involved in measuring the planum and other brain structures using MRI, and by also using functional neuroimaging techniques to examine brain functions in reading and language disabled children.

The paper by Steinmetz and Galaburda focuses on the anatomic definition of the planum temporale on MRI scans, and discusses some of the problems with viewing planum symmetry *per se* as the causative neurological substrate in RD. Because planum symmetry is present in about 25% of neurologically normal individuals, as well as in left handers (only some of both groups being dyslexic), planum symmetry alone cannot be sufficient to produce RD. Other possibilities discussed by these authors include planum symmetry being a co-factor, non-pathological in itself, that limits the ability of the developing brain to compensate for pathological cortical anomalies, or planum symmetry being a consequence or a correlate of other abnormalities in brain development in RD. As the authors imply, twin studies employing both MRI scans and behavioral measures of RD can help to resolve these issues, because such studies can not only determine the heritability of planum symmetry but also the extent of genetic covariation between RD and a brain structure, such as the planum.

In the paper by Hynd, Marshall, and Semrud-Clikeman, previous morphometric work on RD is reviewed, highlighting methodological issues, and the authors own work on brain structure in RD is presented. Besides alterations in planum symmetry, these authors have also found a smaller bilateral insular length and symmetrical frontal regions in RD. They included an important control group in their studies, non-dyslexic ADHD children, to address the issue of discriminant validity of the MRI findings in RD. They have also begun the important task of statistically testing relations between brain structures and brain functions, as measured by neuropsychological tests. These neurolinguistic relationships extend beyond the planum and other posterior language structures. Again, in this paper there is an emphasis that a single localized alteration in brain morphology, such as planum symmetry, is unlikely to be sufficient to produce RD, and that instead we need to think of a pattern of alterations across several connected cortical zones.

This emphasis on a distributed pattern of brain alterations is carried even further in the next paper by Tallal, Sainburg and Jernigan, which examined brain structure and function in developmental language disorder (DLD). Using MRI scans, they performed volumetric analyses of cortical *and* subcortical grey matter. They found bilateral volume reductions in DLD children relative to controls in the posterior peri-sylvian region (which includes the planum temporale), as well as subcortical volume reductions in the right diencephalon and caudate. Symmetry differences were found in the prefrontal and superior parietal/parietal — occipital regions. In the former, anterior region, DLDs exhibited a $L < R$ asymmetry, whereas controls were symmetrical; in the latter, posterior region, DLDs had $L > R$ asymmetry, whereas controls had a $R > L$ pattern. These results are somewhat different than those found in RD, but it is important to remember that this study used both a different population and different morphometric definitions. These authors also review their programmatic work indicating a basic temporal processing deficit in DLD and offer two interesting theories for relating the structural and behavioral data.

The fourth paper by Wood, Flowers, and Buchsbaum reviews their work using three different physiologic measures of brain function in RD, regional cerebral blood flow (rCBF), positron emission tomography (PET), and auditory evoked responses (AERs). Techniques such as these provide an important, intervening level of analysis between studies of brain structure on the one hand and studies of behavior on the other. Structural differences do not necessarily lead to behavioral differences; even when they do, we are still uncertain about intervening mechanisms. What we would like to know is how a change in structure affects the neural computations that eventuate in complex behaviors; physiological studies such as these begin to address that issue.

These authors show how converging results from different functional neuroimaging methods, all addressing multiple cortical regions, can begin to illuminate RD alterations in the pattern of temporal lobe functioning during linguistic tasks. In contrast to normals, RDs show effortful, non-automatic processing in the superior left temporal lobe during a phonemic discrimination task; the pattern of correlations between blood flow and task accuracy was negative in normals but positive in RDs. On an orthographic task, dyslexics exhibited a displacement of blood flow from superior temporal lobe to angular gyrus, consistent with a different functional organization of the language cortices in RD. These authors also emphasize the methodological issues raised by their work.

The last two papers use neuropsychological measures to explore RD. Kershner and Micallef use directed attention dichotic listening to explore both speech lateralization in dysphonetic dyslexics and how "over-functioning" of right hemisphere spatial attentional mechanisms could disrupt left hemisphere phonological processes. Unlike Orton's prediction, these authors did not find altered lateralization for speech perception in dyslexics. But they did find that, within the dyslexic group, right hemisphere attentional activation correlated *negatively* with pseudoword decoding. The authors speculate that a larger right planum may be the structural basis of this right hemisphere attentional "interference" with phonological processing.

The paper by Aguiar and Brady used a clever experiment to further specify the basis of vocabulary differences between RD and normal children. They were able to show that these differences appear to be attributable to differences in the acquisition of the phonological labels for new words and not to other possible processes, such as retention of the conceptual or semantic information in new words. A problem in learning phonological labels could easily result from the left temporal lobe structural and functional anomalies identified in the other papers in this section.

In summary, anatomical differences in dyslexic brains are not confined to a single localization, but instead affect a distributed network of cortical (and possible subcortical) sites involved in language (and possibly attentional) processing. These alterations lead to a processing architecture that is both less efficient at certain linguistic tasks (especially phonological ones) and qualitatively different in the way it handles such tasks. Obviously more work is needed to integrate the findings from different laboratories in this new area of investigation, but the convergence at a broad level is encouraging. It is also clear that such studies hold the additional promise of providing fundamental insights about how brain organization is related to the neural computations necessary for language.

Discussion

There are two papers in this section, one by Alvin Liberman and the other by John Stein. They not only address the previous papers, but also each other. Liberman's paper elegantly explains the apparent paradox that reading is difficult *because* speech is easy. He also explains why inherited differences in the metalinguistic skill of phoneme awareness are to be expected, even though speech itself is species-typical.

Stein, in turn, addresses himself to an issue raised by Liberman — why is there no evidence for a visual linguistic module? He argues for a contribution of right hemisphere spatial and attentional processes to RD, while maintaining that these processes do not constitute a visual linguistic module. He also argues that genetic influences on RD are influences not on reading *per se* or even on spoken language processes, but instead on hemispheric specialization. He further argues that these alterations in hemispheric specialization affect both linguistic *and* visual processes. This is a provocative argument, and represents an alternative perspective to the now mainstream view that RD is mainly a phonological disorder.

In closing, I hope this overview provides a roadmap to the rich territory that follows. Obviously there are many nuances, complexities, and important issues that I have not been able to include here, and which readers must discover for themselves. My fondest wishes for the volume are that it will stimulate new research that will fill in the gaps in our emerging neuroscientific understanding of RD, and that it will also help practitioners better understand and treat the many children *and* adults with this disorder.

ACKNOWLEDGMENTS

First of all, I would like to thank my administrative assistant, Deborah Porter, for all her special efforts in organizing the Rodin Conference and in helping to edit this volume. I would also like to thank John DeFries, James Duncan, Jeffrey Gilger, Richard Olson, and James Stevenson for their help in reviewing manuscripts, and Malatesha Joshi for his encouragement of this special volume. During the preparation of this volume, I was supported by a NIMH RSDA (MH00419), a NIMH MERIT (MH38820), and a NICHD Center Grant (HD27802), as well as by grants from the March of Dimes (12-227) and the Orton Dyslexia Society.

REFERENCES

Clark, D. B. 1988. *Dyslexia: Theory and practice of remedial instruction*. Parkton, MD: York Press.

Galaburda, A. M. and Kemper, T. L. 1979. Cytoarchitetonic abnormalities in developmental dyslexia: A case study. *Annals of Neurology, 6*, 94—100.

Galaburda, A. M., Sherman, G. F., Rosen, G. D., Aboitiz, F., and Geschwind, N. 1985. Developmental dyslexia: Four consecutive patients with cortical anomalies. *Annals of Neurology, 18*, 222—233.

Greenough, W. T., Black, J. E., and Wallace, C. S. 1987. Experience and brain development. *Child Development, 58*, 539—559.

Hynd, G. W., Semrud-Clikeman, M., Lorys, A. R., Novey, E. S., and Eliopulos, D. 1990. Brain morphology in developmental dyslexia and attention deficit disorder/hyperactivity. *Archives of Neurology, 47*, 919—926.

Larsen, J. P., Hoien, T., Lundberg, I., and Odegaard, H. 1990. MRI evaluation of the size and symmetry of the planum temparale in adolescents with developmental dyselxia. *Brain and Language, 39*, 289—301.

Lefly, D. L. and Pennington, B. F. (in press). Spelling errors and reading fluency in compensated adult dyslexics. *Annals of Dyslexia.*

Pennington, B. F., Gilger, J., Pauls, D., Smith, S. A., Smith, S. D., and DeFries, J. C. (in press). Evidence for major gene transmission of developmental dyslexia. *Journal of the American Medical Association.*

Scarr, S. and McCartney, K. 1983. How people make their own environments: A theory of genotype-environment effects. *Child Development, 54,* 424—435.

Shaywitz, S. E., Shaywitz, B. A., Fletcher, J. M., and Escobar, M. D. 1990. Prevalence of reading disabilities in boys and girls: Results of the Connecticut Longitudinal Study. *Journal of the American Medical Association, 265,* 998—1002.

Smith, S. D., Kimberling, W. J., Pennington, B. F., and Lubs, H. A. 1983. Specific reading disability: Identification of an inherited form through linkage analysis. *Science, 219,* 1345—1347.

Genetics

Risk for Reading Disability as a Function of Parental History in Three Family Studies

JEFFREY W. GILGER,[1] BRUCE F. PENNINGTON [2] and J. C. DEFRIES[3]

[1] *University of Denver*; [2] *University of Denver*; [3] *University of Colorado*

ABSTRACT: Inverse Bayesian analyses were applied to data from three large family studies of reading disability to estimate the posterior probability that an offspring will be affected, given that a parent reported a history of learning problems. Prior analyses presented elsewhere (Pennington et al., 1990), suggest that family transmission in these three studies is consistent with major gene or polygene influence. Posterior probability rates are presented in this paper for male to female sex ratios of 3.5:1 and 1:1, with population incidences estimated at 0.05 and 0.10. Results indicate that offspring risk rates are significantly elevated if a parent reports a history of RD. Specifically, an offspring's risk was increased 2 to 80 times over population expectancies when there was an affected parent. While the posterior probabilities and relative risk rates were fairly similar across studies, there was also some variation, which may reflect the different genetic mechanisms operating in these families. This study concludes that both absolute and relative risks are sufficiently increased in families with RD parents to warrant use of family history as a component in clinical evaluation. It is also evident from these results that consideration of the apparent mode of genetic transmission in families may provide even better information as to offspring risk, when family history is obtained.

KEYWORDS: Reading disability, genetics, Bayesian probability, risk, history.

Several pre, peri, and post-natal factors have been shown to place a child at risk for developing a learning disability (Schulman and Leviton, 1978; Dworkin, 1985; Satz and Friel, 1974; Satz, Taylor, Friel, and Fletcher, 1978; Lewis, 1980; DeRuiter, Ferrell, and Kass, 1975; Wissink, Kass, and Ferrell, 1975). Included among these risk factors is a family history of learning problems (Pennington and Smith, 1988). In clinical practice it is commonly observed that a child patient may have other family members who also have learning difficulties. Frequently, a parent will report multiple generations where the patient's relatives had difficulty in reading or spelling, even as adults. Thus it appears that family history may be among the important risk factors in the development of a learning disorder. This conclusion is also suggested by the family and twin studies showing a heritable component to learning disabilities (Pennington and Smith, 1988).

Using data from the Colorado Family Reading Study (DeFries and Decker, 1982; DeFries, Vogler, and LaBuda, 1986), Vogler, DeFries and

Reading and Writing: An Interdisciplinary Journal **3**: 205—217, 1991.
© 1991 *Kluwer Academic Publishers.*

Decker (1985) examined how a child's risk for being reading disabled was modified by the presence of parental self-report history for reading problems. Using inverse Bayesian probability, the increase of risk was anywhere from approximately 4 to 13 times larger if a child had a parent affected according to history, than if the parent reported no history of reading difficulties. The authors concluded that the increase in risk as a function of parental history was high enough to warrant incorporation into a clinical protocol.

For a condition such as reading disability (RD), where genetic influence has been implicated, the probability that an affected parent's offspring will also be affected depends on a number of factors. One of these factors is the type of genetic mechanism involved. For instance, in a condition where there is a completely dominant, fully expressed gene acting, and one parent is affected, we expect, on average, at least 50% of the offspring to also be affected. In the case where many different genes, or polygenes, contribute equally to the condition, such that a certain number of these genes are required for an offspring to be affected, the probability of the condition being expressed in offspring is more difficult to predict, though it is probably less than 50%. The reason why the inheritance patterns of polygenic conditions are more difficult to define precisely, is that they depend more heavily on the genetic make-up of both parents, and which alleles or genes an offspring inherits from either parent, and how these alleles may interact.

We have recently completed complex genetic segregation analyses on four data sets, including the Colorado Family Reading Study, where families were ascertained through an RD adult or child (Pennington, Gilger, Pauls, Smith, Smith, and DeFries, 1990). Three of these data sets yielded results consistent with what would be expected if a single gene was contributing to the transmission of reading disorders in these families. Although major gene influence was not evident in the fourth data set, multi-factorial/polygenic influence appeared to be a significant contributor to the familiality of reading problems. It is noteworthy, that in the three data sets manifesting apparent major gene influence, estimates of the magnitude of the genetic effect, the disease threshold, gene frequency, and sex-dependent penetrances, were all very similar. Genetic heterogeneity is still possible however, and similar parameter estimates across these data sets does not prove that the same gene is operating.

In this paper we repeat the Bayesian analyses of Vogler, DeFies, and Decker (1985) on these data sets, with three major objectives in mind: First, we will examine how, and if, the risk estimates vary across the samples, and how these estimates compare to those reported by Vogler et al. (1985). Second, we will examine whether or not any variability in these estimates is tied to differences in the type of genetic mechanism (polygenic versus major gene) implicated in these families. And third, we will present posterior probabilities based on calculations representing the upper (3.5:1) and lower (1:1) bounds of the estimated male to female sex ratio for RD in the population. Rates for the two sex ratios will be given for comparison purposes. Where it was once believed that RD males substantially outnumbered RD females, some recent studies have in fact demonstrated that, after controlling for selection biases, the actual sex ratio may approach unity (DeFries, Olson, Pennington, Smith, 1990; Shaywitz, Shaywitz, Fletcher, and Escobar, 1990).

METHOD

Three out of the four family data sets were of sufficient size to be included in this paper: The Iowa Family Study of Reading Disabilities (Gilger, 1990a), the reading disabled families from the linkage work of Smith, Pennington, and colleagues (Smith et al., 1983; Pennington et al., 1984), and data from the Colorado Family Reading Study (DeFries and Decker, 1982; DeFries, Vogler, and LaBuda, 1986) which were also used in the Vogler et al. report. Each sample was ascertained in a different manner from different populations, and the individual methodologies are summarized below.

The Iowa Study

Subjects. As part of an ongoing study of dyslexia, data have been gathered for three generations of 40 families selected through a dyslexic proband seen at the University of Iowa Pediatric Psychology Clinic. Dyslexic probands met the inclusionary and exclusionary criteria detailed in DSM III (American Psychiatric Association, 1987). A further requirement was that all probands demonstrated the "memory deficit" subtype of the University of Iowa diagnostic scheme (Richman, 1983; Lindgren, Richman, and Eliason, 1986). Children possessing the memory subtype are distinguishable from other reading disabled children by their characteristic pattern of memory deficits and largely normal functioning in general intelligence, perceptual-motor skills, and associative reasoning. Specifically, in addition to the classic symptoms of dyslexia, the memory disordered group demonstrates the following characteristics: 1. A verbal IQ within 11 points of their Performance IQ; 2. A Verbal and Performance IQ of at least 90; 3. Scores at least 1 standard deviation below average on more than one memory test (e.g., short or long term verbal and visual memory tests), while showing no deficits in associative reasoning and visuo-perceptual skills. All index cases were between 9 and 18 years of age at the time they were seen in the pediatrics clinic.

Subsequent to identifying an appropriate proband, the participation of relatives was solicited through the mail, and followed-up by telephone. All proband siblings, aunts, uncles, grandparents, and cousins in affected kindreds were asked to take part in the study. Thus far data have been collected for approximately 660 individuals of these RD kindreds. Data on a set of control probands (matched to affected probands on SES, grade, sex and age), and their immediate families have also been collected. Though appropriate matches for all affected probands have not yet been obtained, data are available on approximately 500 individuals from these control families.

Materials and RD Diagnosis. As part of the study, adult subjects complete questionnaires at home and return them by mail. Brief telephone interviews are also conducted. Topics addressed by the surveys pertain to aspects of the respondent's physical and socio-emotional development, and the presence of symptoms suggestive of learning disabilities and behavioral disorders. Adequate validity and reliability of self and parent reports has been demonstrated for a variety of the questionnaire items used in the Iowa study (Gilger, Geary, and Eisele, 1990; Gilger, 1990b).

Archival objective test data (national and state percentile scores) are also obtained for the probands, their siblings, cousins, aunts, uncles, and parents. Such data are made available through the University of Iowa Testing Program, which has maintained extensive records of the Iowa Tests of Basic Skills since their inception in the early 1940s (Hieronymus and Hoover, 1986; Iowa Testing Program, 1987). We have attempted to collect at least one set of scores representing the elementary school years (3rd—8th grades) and at least one set from the high school years for all subjects.

For the purposes of this paper, subjects were classified as either RD or not reading disabled (NRD) through an algorithm using the survey data. Probands and their parents were diagnosed as RD by history (i.e. ever having had special education, difficulty in learning while in school, poor academic achievement in the 1st through 3rd, 4th through 8th, or 9th through 12th grades). These questions and positive responses to them, were found to adequately discriminate between the RD and NRD matched control probands.

The Linkage Kindreds

Subjects. Over ten years ago a collaborative study was begun that was aimed at conducting a linkage analysis of families selected through a dyslexic proband (Smith et al., 1983; Smith et al., 1986). All probands were ascertained through clinics or referred from clinic sources, and only those pedigrees suggestive of autosomal, major gene transmission (e.g., a three-generation history of familial reading problems) of dyslexia were asked to participate. Thus far, data on approximately 330 subjects from 21 three-generation kindreds have been obtained. Mean proband age in years is 18.9, with a standard deviation of 8.9.

Materials and RD Diagnosis. Subjects were tested and interviewed by trained personnel, though in some cases family members were either unable or unwilling to complete the study. A battery of tests and questionnaires were given to child and adult subjects, and blood samples were taken. Among the surveys was a handedness inventory and a Reading History survey (Finnucci, Isaacs, and Whitehouse, 1982). Medical, socio-emotional, and other general information was also obtained.

Subjects are diagnosed as RD if they report having had a history of reading problems on the Reading History Survey. On the rare occasion that self-report history data was not available, a subject may have been diagnosed as RD if person-to-person interviews with the subject, or information from a blood relative positively indicated reading difficulties.

The Colorado Family Reading Study

Subjects. Subjects were referred for the study by personnel of the Boulder Valley and St. Vrain Valley school districts in Colorado. All probands had IQ's of 90 or above; reading achievement level of one half, or lower, of grade expectancy; chronological age between 7.5 and 12 years; resided with both biological parents; met the exclusionary criteria of DSM III (e.g., no uncorrected visual deficits, no emotional impairments, etc.). Control children were matched to reading-disabled children on the basis of age (within 6 months), sex, grade, school, and neighborhood. Except for reading level, which was normal or above, the controls met the criteria used for the ascertainment of affected probands. In addition to the index cases, data were obtained on the parents and siblings of control and affected families. Data are currently available on approximately 565 individuals from 133 nuclear families selected through a reading disabled child.

Materials and RD Diagnosis. All subjects received an extensive 2—3 hour test battery which included measures of intelligence, academic skills, and specific cognitive abilities. Parental self-report and parent-child report survey information was also obtained on topics related to current and past academic, medical, and socio-emotional status.

RD diagnosis for this paper is the same as for the earlier Vogler et al. study. Specifically, subjects were classified as RD if they responded positively to a single question addressing serious difficulty in learning to read.

ANALYSES

The ideal way to estimate the risk of being an affected offspring is to ascertain affected and unaffected groups of parents, and examine the frequency with which the children are affected with RD. However, family studies, such as the ones reported herein, are typically retrospective in nature, where the affection status of parents is determined after the family has been ascertained through an affected child. Thus, we cannot directly calculate the offspring probability of being RD, given that a parent is RD. An indirect method however, using an inverse Bayesian probability formula, does provide a means of estimating the likelihood a child will be affected given that the parental reading status is known.

The posterior probability that a child will be affected [P(C/R)], given that a parent is affected, can be found by the following equation (Winkler, 1972):

$$P(C/R) = \frac{P(C)P(R/C)}{P(C)P(R/C) + P(\text{Not } C)P(R/\text{Not } C)}$$

The parameters in the above equation are defined as follows: P(C) = the prior probability that a child will be RD, or an estimate of the population incidence; P(Not C) = 1 − P(C), or the likelihood that a child will not be RD; P(R/C) = the probability that a parent will be RD given that a child is RD, a value determined from the incidence of RD among parents of probands; P(R/C not C) = the probability that a parent will be RD given that the child is not RD, a value ascertained from the incidence of RD in parents of controls; P(C/R) = the posterior likelihood that a child will be RD given the parental affection status.

For this paper we followed a methodology similar to Vogler, DeFries and Decker (1985). First, we used two estimates of the population base rate for RD: 0.05, and 0.10 percent. We then used these rates to calculate P(C) separately for each sex, assuming a male to female sex ratio of 3.5:1, and again for a ratio of 1:1. Second, P(R/C) was calculated separately for mothers and fathers, and further subdivided by the sex of the proband. Finally, P(R/Not C) was obtained from the Colorado Family study control parents, and as noted in the Vogler et al. paper, 4% of the control fathers, and 3% of the control mothers reported a history of reading problems. There were essentially no differences in parental affection rates as a function of the sex of the proband. Since the Iowa control families were not all adequately matched to Iowa RD families, their data were not used in the P(R/Not C) estimates.

In the analyses that follow, only the proband nuclear families were used. In the case of the Iowa and Linkage samples, nuclear families other than those of the probands (e.g., cousins) were available. We did not use these additional families because of ambiguity in defining a child proband from each, and a desire for consistency across the three samples, where only proband nuclear family data was always available. Moreover, only those nuclear families where diagnostic data were available for both parents were used. Thus, in some cases the N sizes may deviate slightly from those reported elsewhere in this paper.

RESULTS

Table 1 shows the probability of a mother or father being affected given affected or control offspring [P(R/C) and P(R/Not C)]. Several aspects of the data in Table 1 are noteworthy. First, there is some variability in the parental probabilities across the three studies. Estimates are most similar for the father affection status of male probands, and the mother affection status of female probands. Second, the rates of RD in the parents of RD probands are clearly elevated over population base rates (e.g., 0.05, and 0.10), and over the rates found in controls as well. Third, there are minor differences between the rates we report for the Colorado study and those reported by Vogler et al. This is a consequence of the differences in the

Table 1. Parental affection status of male and female RD and control probands[a]

	N	RD Father	NRD Father	RD Mother	NRD Mother
Iowa Study:					
Male Probands	26	0.35	0.65	0.12	0.88
Female Probands	12	0.17	0.83	0.42	0.58
Linkage Study:					
Male Probands	15	0.53	0.47	0.67	0.33
Female Probands	6	0.83	0.17	0.33	0.67
Colorado Study:					
Male Probands	99	0.30	0.70	0.15	0.85
Female Probands	27	0.41	0.59	0.30	0.70
Controls	182	0.04	0.96	0.03	0.97

[a] RD = Reading Disabled; NRD = Normal.

sample. On the other hand, there is a tendency for the smallest estimates to come from the Iowa sample. Specifically, the Iowa data set gave the smallest probabilities for 5 out of the 8 possible within child-sex and parent-sex comparisons. While small sample sizes mandate cautious interpretation of these data, they are somewhat consistent with the hypothesis of major (dominant or semi-dominant) gene influence in the Colorado, and especially the Linkage families, and polygenic inheritance in kindreds from Iowa. It is also noteworthy however, that the relative risk estimates and posterior probabilities of the Iowa and Colorado data sets are quite similar in magnitude.

Finally, the Colorado analyses of Vogler et al. indicated that the absolute risk for female offspring was smaller than that for males, though the female relative risk was roughly 1/2 to 2 1/2 times larger, depending on the population incidence used. While the relative risk estimates derived from the current Colorado data reflect this same trend, the Iowa and Linkage data do not for either of the two sex ratios used. For the Iowa sample, relative risks were higher for females only if the mother was RD, and in the Linkage sample, females demonstrated higher risks only if they had an RD father. However, for all three samples, the *average* relative risk estimates were larger for female offspring.

DISCUSSION

In general the results reported in this paper indicate that there is a substantial increase in the childhood risk for RD given an affected parent. Though there were some inconsistencies across studies of the posterior probability estimates, given the vast differences in the diagnostic criteria, design, and populations used in the studies, it is surprising how similar the pattern of results actually were, especially for the Iowa and Colorado samples. Some of the variability observed may reflect parameter instability due to the relatively small number of Iowa and Linkage proband nuclear families. Nonetheless, similar to Vogler, DeFries and Decker (1985), the data we report suggest that consideration of family (parental) history of reading problems may add important information pertinent to the diagnosis and prediction of reading disabilities in children. Our results show that using family data in conjunction with other risk indicators may provide a powerful diagnostic and predictive tool in future clinical and experimental work.

All three projects, particularly the Iowa and Linkage studies, are subject to the response biases prevalent among clinically ascertained or referred samples, and this may have artificially inflated the posterior probabilities and relative risk estimates obtained. While only the Linkage study purposely ascertained families having three or more generations of affected individuals, it has been our experience that there is a bias towards multiplex families participating in research of this type in general. Therefore, the risk estimates we provide probably represent the upper limits of the "true" probabilities of affection given knowledge of parental reading ability, since our families may have a higher than average genetic loading, or a priori probability towards having RD offspring. Furthermore, it is important to bear in mind that even minor modifications of the population incidence, P(C), or estimated affection rates in control samples, P(R/Not C), can have large effects on the posterior probabilities obtained. In this report we used the same control sample and P(R/Not C) estimates when calculating P(C/R) for all three data sets. Thus, in a sense, the results across data sets are not completely independent. Separate and appropriately matched and identified control samples for each family study may have altered our posterior probabilities. However, confidence can be placed in using the only Colorado control sample, given that P(R/Not C) estimates approximated those we'd expect given general population base rates.

Relative risk estimates seemed higher than expected, particularly for the Linkage sample, and there was a tendency for the lowest risks to come from the Iowa data set. Recall that polygenic factors have been implicated in RD transmission in the Iowa pedigrees, whereas the Colorado and Linkage data sets show major (dominant or semi-dominant) gene influence according to our segregation analyses (Pennington et al., 1990). Therefore, the lower rates in the Iowa sample are in accordance with expectancy.

In summary, the results presented in this paper indicate that parental affection status has a profound impact on the likelihood that offspring will express a reading disorder. The data also suggest that the probability of being affected may vary in response to genetic heterogeneity, or differing modes of genetic transmission operating within families. There is also some evidence that complex sex effects may be operating that alter the posterior probabilities that a child will have RD. Future work, perhaps with different potential predictors of offspring risk, should involve incorporating the mode of genetic transmission into predictive risk models, as well as the parent and offspring sex. This will of course require a better understanding of the genetics and mechanisms behind RD inheritance and expression than is currently available.

AUTHOR NOTES

Address reprint requests to the first author at the University of Denver, Department of Psychology, Frontier Hall, 2155 S. Race Street, Denver, CO, 80208. The authors wish to thank the families who participated in the studies, as well as Drs. Ray Crowe, Lynn Richman and H. D. Hoover of the University of Iowa. Portions of this paper were presented at the Rodin Foundation conference on Genetic and Neurological Influences on Dyslexia, Boulder, CO, September, 1990.

During preparation of this article Dr. Gilger was supported in part, by a Fellowship in Developmental Psychobiology through the University of Colorado (MH15442). Dr. Pennington was supported by a NIMH RSDA (MH00419), project grant (MH38820), and grants from the March of Dimes (12-135) and the Orton Dyslexia Society. The Colorado Family Reading Study was funded in part by grants from the Spencer Foundation, NICHD (HD-11681), and NIMH (MH-16880) to Dr. DeFries. During collection of the Iowa Family data, Dr. Gilger was funded by a training fellowship in Psychiatric Genetics at the University of Iowa Medical School (#MH146201-13 12).

REFERENCES

American Psychiatric Association. 1987. *Diagnostic and statistical manual of mental disorders* (3rd edition-Revised). Washington D.C.: APA Press.

DeFries, J. C., Olson, R. K., Pennington, B. F., and Smith, S. D. 1991. The Colorado Reading Project: An update. In D. B. Gray and D. Duane (Eds.), *The reading brain: The biological basis of dyslexia.* Parkton, MA.: York Press.

DeFries, J. C. and Decker, S. 1982. Genetic aspects of reading disability: A family study. In R. N. Malatesha and P. G. Aaron (Eds.), *Reading disorders: Varieties and treatments.* New York: Academic Press.

DeFries, J. C., Vogler, G. P., and LaBuda, M. 1986. Colorado Family Reading Study: An overview. In J. Fuller and E. Simmel (Eds.), *Perspectives in behavior genetics, Principles and Application II*, Hillsdale, N.J.

DeRuiter, J. A., Ferrell, W. R., and Kass, C. E. 1975. Learning disability classification by Bayesian aggregation of test results. *Journal of Learning Disabilities, 8*, 365—372.

Dworkin, P. H. 1985. *Learning and behavior problems of school children.* Philadelphia, PA: W.B. Saunders Co.

Finnuci, J. M., Isaacs, S. D., Whitehouse, C. C., and Childs, B. 1982. Empirical validation of reading and spelling quotients. *Developmental Medicine and Child Neurology, 24*, 733—744.

Gilger, J. W. 1990a. *Reading disorders in families: Genetics and developement.* Unpublished manuscript.

Gilger, J. W. 1990b. Using self-report and parental-report data to assess past and present academic achievement of adults and children. Submitted for review.

Gilger, J. W., Geary, D. C., and Eisele, L. 1990. Reliability and validity of retrospective self-reports of pubertal events using twin, sibling, and college student data. *Adolescence*, In press.

Hieronymous, A. N. and Hoover, H. D. 1986. *Manual for school administrators for the ITBS.* Chicago, Ill: Riverside Publishing Co.

Iowa Testing Program 1987. *Manual for teachers, administrators and counselors for the ITED.* Iowa City, IA: The University of Iowa.

Lewis, A. 1980. The early identification of children with learning difficulties. *Journal of Learning Disabilities, 13*, 102—108.

Lindgren, S. D., Richman, L., and Eliason, M. 1986. Memory processes in reading disability subtypes. *Developmental Neuropsychology, 2*, 173—181.

Pennington, B. F., Gilger, J. W., Pauls, D., Smith, S. A., Smith, S. D., and DeFries, J. C. 1990. Segregation analyses of four samples of dylsexic families. Submitted for review.

Pennington, B. F. and Smith, S. D. 1988. Genetic influences on learning disabilities: An update. *Journal of Consulting and Clinical Psychology, 56*, 817—823.

Pennington, B. F., Smith, S. D., McCable, L. L., Kimberling, W. J., and Lubs, H. A. 1984.

Developmental continuities and discontinuities in a form of familial dyslexia. In R. Emde and R. Harman (Eds.), *Continuities and discontinuities in development* (pp. 123—151). New York: Plenum Press.
Richman, L. 1983. Language-Learning Disability: Issues, research, and future directions. *Advances in Developmental and Behavioral Pediatrics, 4*, 87—107.
Satz, P. and Friel, J. 1974. Some predictive antecedents of specific reading disability: A preliminary two-year follow-up. *Journal of Learning Disabilities, 7*, 437—444.
Satz, P., Taylor, H. G., Friel, J., and Fletcher, J. 1978. Some development and predictive precursors of reading disabilities: A six year follow-up. In A. L. Benton and D. Pearl (Eds.), *Dyslexia: An appraisal of current knowledge* (pp. 313—348). New York: Oxford University Press.
Schulman, J. and Leviton, A. 1978. Reading disabilities: An epidemiologic approach. In H. R. Mykelbust (Ed.), *Progress in learning disabilities* (vol. 4, pp. 65—96). New York: Grune & Stratton.
Shaywitz, S. E., Shaywitz, B. A., Fletcher, J. M., and Escobar, M. D. 1990. Prevalence of reading disabilities in boys and girls: Results of the Connecticut Longitudinal Study. *Journal of the American Medical Association, 264*(8), 998—1002.
Smith, S. D., Kimberling, W. J., Pennington, B., and Lubs, H. A. 1983. Specific reading disability: Identification of an inherited form through linkage analysis. *Science, 219*, 1345—1347.
Smith, S. D., Pennington, B. F., Kimberling, W. J., Fain, P. R., Ing, P. S., and Lubs, H. A. 1986. Genetic heterogeneity in specific reading disability. *American Journal of Human Genetics, 39*, A169.
Vogler, G. P., DeFries, J. C., and Decker, S. 1985. Family history as an indicator of risk for reading disability. *Journal of Learning Disabilities, 18*, 419—421.
Winkler, R. L. 1972. *Introduction to Bayesian inference and decision.* New York: Holt, Rinehart & Winston.
Wissink, J., Kass, C. E., and Ferrell, W. R. 1975. A Bayesian approach to the identification of children with learning disabilities. *Journal of Learning Disabilities, 8*, 158—166.

Antecedents to Reading Disability: Preschool Language Development and Literacy Experiences of Children from Dyslexic Families

HOLLIS S. SCARBOROUGH

Department of Psychology
Brooklyn College — City University of New York
Brooklyn, NY 11210

ABSTRACT: In a longitudinal study of the relation between preschool development and later reading abilities, children with dyslexic parents and/or older siblings were compared to children with no family incidence of dyslexia. Many children from dyslexic families developed reading problems by the end of the second grade, and these poor readers were characterized chiefly by weaker early syntactic and phonological skills and by less frequent exposure to books during their preschool years than the preschoolers who became normal readers. Some implications of the results for etiological theories of dyslexia are discussed.

KEYWORDS: Development, dyslexia, emergent literacy, language, phonology, reading disability, speech, syntax.

How do dyslexic children differ from nondyslexic children early in life, *before* they have been taught anything about reading and writing? What do such early differences tell us about the neurocognitive underpinnings of dyslexia? Are the early literacy-related experiences of dyslexic children different from those of other children? If so, how might such experiential differences interact with a child's genetic endowment in the etiology of dyslexia? Questions like these are being addressed in the longitudinal prospective study to be described here. Although final answers cannot yet be provided, the results to date suggest some interesting hypotheses about the nature and developmental course of dyslexia.

OVERVIEW OF THE STUDY: SAMPLING, DATA COLLECTION, AND OUTCOME DETERMINATIONS

Starting in 1980, observations were made of the preschool development of a sample of 78 children from middle-class families residing in central New Jersey.[1] During visits to the subjects' homes at ages 24, 30, 36, 42, 48 and 60 months, a variety of cognitive and linguistic tests was administered, behavior in several observational contexts was videorecorded, and ques-

Reading and Writing: An Interdisciplinary Journal 3: 219—233, 1991.
© 1991 *Kluwer Academic Publishers.*

dyslexic families are nearly equivalent in the percentage of their family members with reading problems: 57.1% vs. 53.3%, respectively. The *Control* group consists of 22 of the children from nondyslexic families who became normal readers. They were selected so as to resemble the Dyslexic group as closely as possible with respect to SES, IQ, and sex; the normal readers who were not included are generally higher-SES, higher-IQ girls (Scarborough, 1990b).

The Dyslexic and Control groups will be compared to address questions about early developmental differences that precede and may contribute to later reading achievement differences. The Dyslexic and Family groups, on the other hand, will be compared to address questions about the effects of being raised in a dyslexic family on the development of good versus poor verbal skills.

PRESCHOOL ANTECEDENTS OF READING PROBLEMS

Language and Preliteracy Skills at Age Five

Several potential predictors of subsequent reading achievement were assessed at age 60 months: IQ, visual discrimination, story comprehension, picture naming speed, picture naming accuracy, letter identification, knowledge of letter-sound correspondences, and phonemic awareness. Of these, only the latter four were related to outcome reading status (Scarborough, 1989; 1990b). These results, first of all, replicate many prior prospective findings demonstrating the importance of language and preliteracy abilities during the late preschool years as predictors of subsequent reading achievement (e.g., Bishop and Adams, in press; Butler, Marsh, Sheppard and Sheppard, 1985; Bryant, Bradley, Maclean and Crossland, 1989; Mann, 1984; Mann and Ditunno, 1990; Share, Jorm, Maclean and Matthews, 1985). Moreover, the fact that the present sample resembles others at this age increases our confidence that our dyslexic children are indeed "typical" disabled readers, and thus that our findings may be generalizable.

The results also confirm that "preliteracy" differences (i.e., differences on tasks that require skills closely associated with reading itself) are well established by this age. As 5-year-olds, the Dyslexic group could identify fewer letters, and were less able to pair pictures with print stimuli on the basis of initial phonemes and graphemes, than could the children in the Family and Control groups. In some sense, therefore, one might say that many children in the Dyslexic group could already be termed "reading disabled," insofar as they were already underachieving in the acquisition of reading. These findings underscore the need to investigate even earlier differences between dyslexic and nondyslexic children, as is the primary focus of the present research project.

Early Language Development

Two kinds of preschool language assessments were obtained for the sample: scores on formal tests of speech discrimination, vocabulary development, and syntax comprehension; and measures derived from naturalistic observations of expressive phonology, vocabulary, and syntax. In general, we have found that the language test scores tend to be correlated with each other and with IQ scores, both concurrently and prospectively, but tend to be less closely related to natural language measures (e.g., Scarborough and Dobrich, 1990). The considerable degree of shared variance among scores on "IQ" and "language" tests undoubtedly arises, in part, from the similar requirements for attending to and cooperating with the examiner, as well as from the similar formats and vocabulary demands of many preschool tests. The critical faculty that underlies dyslexia must be relatively dissociated from general intelligence (Stanovich, 1988), so with respect to identifying this faculty, test scores have rather limited utility. From the outset of this project, therefore, naturalistic observational assessments have been emphasized. As will next be described, those data have provided some interesting insights into the linguistic deficits of dyslexic children.

Several natural language samples were videorecorded during each visit to the child. So far, analyses have been performed on samples from only one observational context: a 30-minute mother-child play session for which all dyads were provided with the same age-appropriate sets of toys. Mothers were instructed to play with their children as they ordinarily would, but to let the child take the lead in choosing what to play with. Each play session was transcribed initially by a trained observer who recorded all maternal and child utterances and relevant contextual notes. This transcript was then reviewed by a more experienced transcriber, whose judgments were accepted when disagreements arose. For 10% to 15% of the play sessions at each age, two transcripts were independently prepared, and then evaluated for the reliability of the transcribers' judgments of the segmentation of speech into utterances and of the morphological and phonemic sequences produced. Percentages of judgments in agreement have typically ranged from 85% to 95%.

To determine whether the children who became disabled readers were indeed deficient in any or all of these facets of language skill, transcripts are first coded for overall syntactic, lexical, and phonological level, yielding four measures: *MLU* (mean length of utterance in morphemes for a sample of 100 child utterances; Brown, 1973), a widely used general indicator of syntactic level; *IPSyn* (Index of Productive Syntax; Scarborough, 1990), a summary score of the syntactic and morphological complexity of a 100-utterance corpus; *Pronunciation Errors*, the number of consonants mispronounced in 100 successive intelligible open-class words; and *Lexical Diversity*, the number of different words within 250 successive word tokens produced by the child (Richards, 1987). (For details see Scarborough, 1990a, 1990b; Scarborough and Dobrich, 1990).

These four expressive language measures were first analyzed for the three contrasted groups at age 30 months (Scarborough, 1990b). At this age, the children in the Control and Family groups, all of whom became normal readers, were highly similar in every respect. In comparison to these children, the 30-month-olds who became disabled readers were deficient in syntactic and phonological, but not lexical, proficiency. These results are consistent with prior prospective findings that older preschool children and kindergartners who develop reading problems exhibit weaknesses in phonological processing (e.g., Bryant et al., 1989; Mann, 1984; Mann and Ditunno, 1990; Share et al., 1985) and syntactic abilities (e.g., Bishop and Adams, in press; Butler et al., 1985).

Further analyses of these data revealed that some unique variance in outcomes was accounted for by early syntactic differences above and beyond that accounted for by the phonological measure, but that the reverse did not obtain (Scarborough, 1990b), suggesting that difficulties with syntactic and morphological aspects of language in the earlier preschool years may be more strongly related to later reading disabilities than were expressive phonological deficits. A follow-up to this intriguing finding was next pursued by computing MLU and IPSyn scores for the Dyslexic and Control groups over the remainder of the preschool period (Scarborough, in press). As shown in Figure 1, the Control group continued to produce longer utterances and more complex syntactic constructions through age 48 months. To determine whether receptive as well as expressive syntactic deficits characterized the Dyslexic group, scores on the Northwestern Syntax Screening Test (NSST; Lee, 1971), which had been given at ages 36, 48, and 60 months, were also analyzed. As illustrated in the figure, the Control group outperformed the Dyslexic group on this test also (even with IQ controlled in the analysis).

At age 60 months, however, there were no longer any group differences on the three syntax measures, indicating that by the time the Dyslexic children were about to enter kindergarten, their syntactic production and comprehension capabilities were no longer seriously impaired. Although they may conceivably have had some subtle residual syntactic deficits that were not detected by our global proficiency measures, it is unlikely that these would have been so severe as to have impeded either their understanding of the relatively simple sentences found in primers or their ability to understand and be understood orally by their teachers.

How, then, were their earlier syntactic problems related to their later reading problems? As noted above, the Dyslexic group was weak in phonemic awareness, naming, and preliteracy knowledge at age 5. Not surprisingly, early expressive syntax abilities were correlated with these later preschool precursors of reading disability (Scarborough, 1990b, in

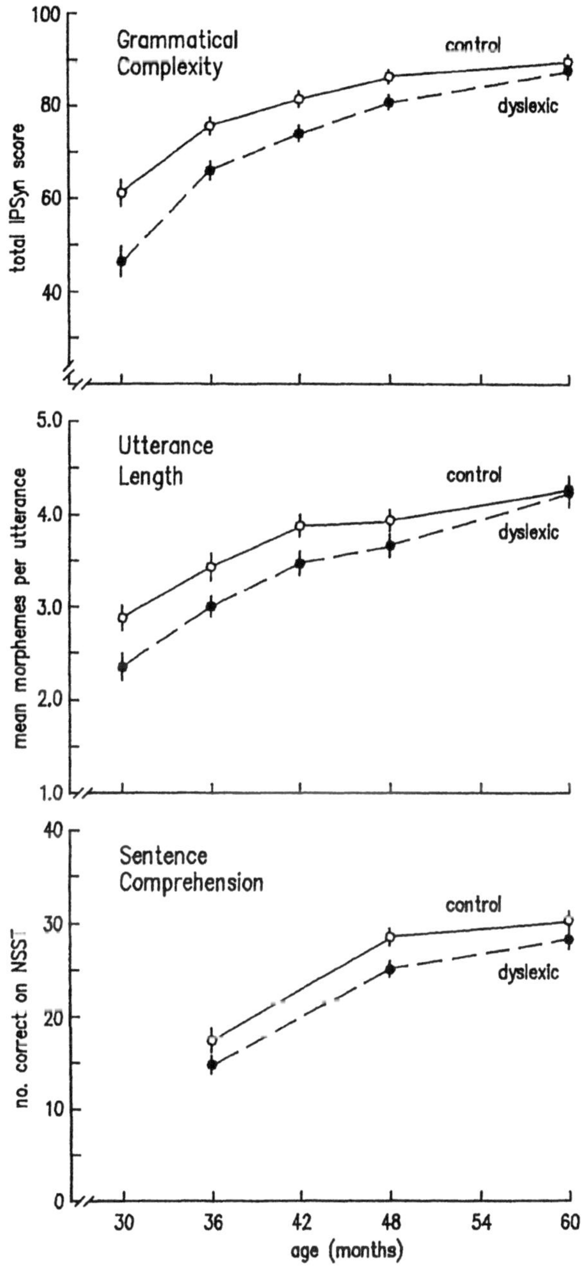

Fig. 1. Preschool development of expressive grammatical complexity, utterance length, and sentence comprehension skills of the Dyslexic and Control groups. Vertical bars extend one standard error above and below the group means at each age.

press). Was the relation of early syntax to eventual reading merely mediated by the intervening differences in phonological processing and literacy-related knowledge, which were actually most responsible for reading disabilities? Apparently not, since a further analysis of IPSyn scores from age 30 to 48 months revealed that even after variance attributable to the 60-months measures was accounted for, the syntactic differences made a unique contribution to outcomes (Scarborough, 1990b, in press).

Consequently, the findings suggest several alternative hypotheses about the relations among developing syntactic, phonological, preliteracy, and reading abilities. First, the fundamental processing problem associated with dyslexia may not be confined to the phonological domain, as is so often hypothesized (e.g., Catts, 1989; Jorm and Share, 1983; Liberman and Shankweiler, 1980; Shankweiler and Crain, 1986; Stanovich, 1988; Wagner and Torgesen, 1987), but rather may involve broader structural language impairments or even more general symbolic rule learning difficulties (e.g., Morrison, 1987). That is, for both syntax and phonology — and for few, if any, other tasks except learning to read — the child must discover and use regularities that govern the order-dependent combination of abstract formal elements into higher-order structures of which only the surface features are uttered and perceived. Any or all of these task demands could conceivably be the source of difficulty for dyslexic children.

Second, the results indicate that the dyslexic child's profile of deficits changes over time, perhaps reflecting the persistent influence of the presumed underlying limitation on the child's responses to a succession of developmental challenges. Such "heterotypic continuity" may characterize many aspects of human cognitive and personality development (Bates, Bretherton and Snyder, 1988; Kagan, 1971; McCall, 1981). For both practical and theoretical reasons, therefore, an increased emphasis on longitudinal research would be valuable for achieving a complete understanding of the nature of dyslexia.

Third, instead of casting the preschool characteristics of dyslexic children as "precursors" and the reading problems of these children as "outcomes," it might be more helpful to view both as successive, observable symptoms of the same condition. I am thus inclined to believe that syntactic limitations per se are *not* largely responsible for the dyslexic child's difficulties in learning to read in any directional or causal sense, but rather that the prediction of the later symptom (reading problems) from an earlier one (syntactic problems) arises because each symptom reflects the same underlying dimension of individual difference. Therefore, while the education goal may be to explain reading difficulty for its own sake, the neuropsychological goal is to define the nature of the fundamental difficulty that manifests itself most evidently, but not solely, as underachievement in reading.

Finally, it must be emphasized that the demonstration of early language deficits in children from dyslexic families who become disabled readers does not, in and of itself, indicate that there is any etiological relation between language development and learning to read. Instead, for instance, the observed language weaknesses might only be correlates of some more important unidentified differences between dyslexic and nondyslexic children. The foregoing hypotheses thus might have to be modified if alternative explanations for the appearance of the various "symptoms" of dyslexia can be established. In the next section, the notion that some early symptoms are a by-product of being raised in a dyslexic family, rather than a result of an intrinsic neurocognitive limitation, will be considered.

EARLY LANGUAGE AND LITERACY EXPERIENCES OF CHILDREN FROM DYSLEXIC FAMILIES

Dyslexic schoolchildren are not only poor readers and spellers, but also have weaker verbal skills and read less often and less avidly than their classmates (e.g., Juel, 1988). These verbal and literacy differences often persist into adolescence and adulthood (e.g., Bruck, 1990; LaBuda and DeFries, 1988). Consequently, children who grow up in households with many such members may be exposed to atypical conditions under which to acquire language and reading skills. The hypothesis that some sort of impoverishment of experience is responsible, in part, for the occurrence or severity of linguistic deficits and reading problems in children from dyslexic families has been addressed in several completed and ongoing analyses.

Maternal Language Input

In the study of language development at age 30 months (Scarborough, 1990b), the children from dyslexic families who became normal readers (Family group) equaled or exceeded the Controls in early syntactic, phonological, and lexical skills as well as in Grade 2 achievement, indicating that familial risk per se did not preclude normal developmental progress. Within the Dyslexic group, furthermore, no differences in language or reading ability were found between the children whose mothers (their primary caretakers and presumed major sources of language input) were disabled readers and those whose mothers were normal readers, again suggesting that the children's syntactic and phonological problems could not readily be attributed to the presumed poorer verbal skills of their early conversational partners. A more definitive test of the hypothesis, in which the quality of maternal speech during the recorded play sessions is evaluated, is now in progress.

Preschool Literacy Experiences

In-home exposure to books and reading during the preschool years is believed to affect children's emerging attitudes and knowledge about literacy (e.g., Teale and Sulzby, 1986; Wells, 1986). In dyslexic families, therefore, youngsters may be exposed to fewer models of adult and parent-child reading, which might impede the growth of reading-related skills and attitudes. In some recent analyses of questionnaire data collected during the preschool phase of this project (Scarborough, Dobrich and Hager, in press), we obtained some evidence that the preschoolers who became disabled readers underwent somewhat different early literacy experiences than the other children. These results are shown in Figure 2, which provides a summary of parental responses to the questions, "How often in a typical week do you and your child read books together?" (asked of the fathers during the intake interview, and of the mothers at each preschool visit through 48 months) and "How often does your child amuse himself/herself alone with books?" (asked of mothers from 36 to 48 months).[4]

Responses to the first question revealed that the Dyslexic group was read to less often by their fathers than were the two groups that became normal readers. For mothers, less joint reading was reported for the Dyslexics than the Controls at age 30 months but not thereafter; there were also marginal differences between the Dyslexic and Family groups at 42 and 48 months but not at the younger ages. In sum, how often the children were read to was not as strongly related to their later reading abilities as has been observed in the more socioculturally diverse Bristol sample (Wells, 1986). On the other hand, in response to the second question, mothers reported observing considerably fewer occurrences of solitary book activity by children in the Dyslexic group than by children in the other groups at all ages.

The parents' questionnaire responses suggest that the children who became disabled readers were typically read to almost daily by their mothers but less than once a week by their fathers, and amused themselves alone with books only 2 or 3 times per week. The preschoolers who became normal readers experienced only slightly more frequent mother-child reading, but were read to several times per week by their fathers and typically engaged in solitary book activity about 5 to 7 times per week. Cumulated over the preschool period, differences of such magnitude may indeed have contributed to the emergence of observed group differences in literacy-related skills by the time the children enter school.

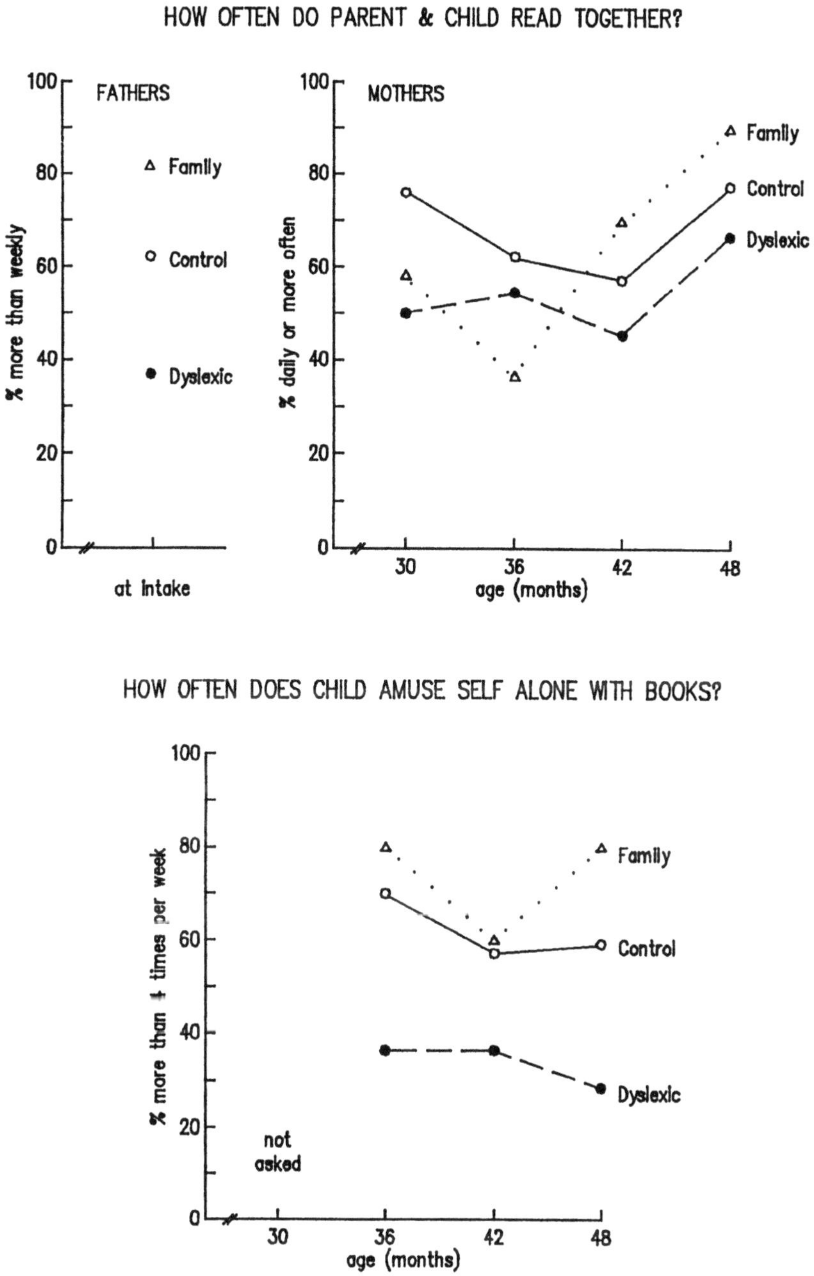

Fig. 2. Summary of responses by parents of the Dyslexic, Family, and Control groups to questions about the children's preschool literacy experiences.

Why was the Dyslexic group exposed to fewer early literacy experiences of this sort? It was originally presumed that dyslexic and nondyslexic parents (and siblings) might provide children with different exposure to books and reading, and these findings are somewhat consistent with that view. Other aspects of the data, however, suggest that the observed differences may instead have been child-driven. First, several parents spontaneously remarked that they read to their children infrequently because the children were not interested in such activity. Second, children in the Dyslexic group were read to less frequently by the *non*dyslexic as well as their dyslexic fathers (42% vs. 30% did so weekly, respectively) and by the *non*dyslexic as well as their dyslexic mothers (56% vs. 50% daily, respectively), suggesting that something about the *children* determined how often their parents read to them. Finally, the reported differences in child-alone book activity did not narrow from 36 to 48 months, as would be expected if cumulated literacy experience (or maturational growth of some sort) were responsible for a child's growing interest in books. Therefore, the hypothesis that intrinsic differences among children in their early interest or disinterest in books may play a role in preschool literacy development — i.e., that the dyslexic children's improverishment of literacy experience may be largely self-imposed — is being addressed in an ongoing analysis of observations of mother-child book-reading that were videorecorded during the preschool phase of this project.

SUMMARY AND IMPLICATIONS

To date, analyses of this longitudinal project have revealed that children with dyslexic parents and older siblings were highly likely to develop reading problems, and that the preschoolers who became disabled readers were characterized primarily by their weak early language abilities (especially syntax) and their infrequent exposure to books (especially in solitary book activities). What are the implications of these results for the focal issues of this volume — the genetic and neurological bases for dyslexia? First, the findings are of interest to behavioral geneticists because they are compatible with, though not proof of, the accumulated evidence for the heritability of reading disabilities. Second, a full understanding of the nature of the dyslexic's cognitive and behavioral limitations would be very helpful, both conceptually and methodologically, for research on genetic and neurological mechanisms. The present results strongly suggest that it would be premature to define the core deficit solely as a phonological one in such studies. Last, the evidence for early disinterest in literacy by children who later became disabled readers may represent a correlation between genetic and experiential factors in early development. The study of such correlations may be necessary to arrive at a complete account of the etiology of dyslexia through the interdisciplinary efforts of behavior geneticists, neuroscientists, and psychologists.

ACKNOWLEDGMENTS

This research has been supported by grants from the National Institute of Child Health and Human Development and the March of Dimes Birth Defects Foundation. The assistance of Wanda Dobrich, Maria Hager, Janet Wyckoff, and many others in the collection and analysis of data is gratefully acknowledged. I would also like to thank the families who participated in the project.

NOTES

[1] The sample originally included 89 children. Ten families discontinued their participation and one child was eliminated because of a clear general developmental disability, leaving 78. All subjects were raised in monolingual English-speaking households, and none had any uncorrected visual, auditory, or neurological impairments.
[2] For the 66 children who were tested by us at Grade 2, reading achievement was assessed with the Reading Cluster of the WJPB (Woodcock and Johnson, 1977). Classifications of the remaining 12 subjects were based on their performance on school administered standardized tests of achievement and aptitude.
[3] Incidence and projected risk rates in other studies (Finucci, Guthrie, Childs, Abbey, and Childs, 1976, Finucci, Gottfredson and Childs, 1985; Gilger, Pennington and DeFries, this volume; Hallgren, 1950; Hoien et al., 1989; Kerns and Decker, 1985; Vogler, DeFries and Decker, 1985; Zahalkova, Vrzal and Kloboukova, 1972) have varied considerably, in part because criteria for defining adult and child reading status have often relied on adults' self reports and children's school classifications, which probably tend to be less reliable than test-based designations (Gilger et al., this volume; Scarborough, 1989; Shaywitz, Shaywitz, Fletcher and Escobar, 1990). When adult self-report and school classifications were used, incidence and risk rates in the present sample were even more similar to those obtained by others than when test scores were used.
[4] Because we were primarily interested in detecting impoverishment of experience, "not at all," "once or twice," "3–4 times," "5–6 times," and "daily or more often" were the maternal response choices offered until 48 months, at which age "daily" and "more than once a day" replaced the previously highest response option for the first question. The fathers were asked an open-ended question, responses to which were coded as "never," "less than once per week," "weekly," "several times per week," and "daily or more often."

REFERENCES

Bates, E., Bretherton, I., and Snyder, L. 1988. *From first words to grammar*. Cambridge: Cambridge University Press.
Bishop, D. V. M. and Adams, C. (in press). A prospective study of the relationship

between specific language impairment, phonological disorders and reading retardation. *Journal of Child Psychology and Psychiatry* (in press).

Brown, R. 1973. *A first language: The early stages*. Cambridge, MA: Cambridge University Press.

Bruck, M. 1990. Word recognition skills of adults with childhood diagnoses of dyslexia. *Developmental Psychology, 26*, 439—454.

Bryant, P. E., Bradley, L., Maclean, M., and Crossland, J. 1989. Nursery rhymes, phonological skills and reading. *Journal of Child Language, 16*, 407—428.

Butler, S. R., Marsh, H. W., Sheppard, M. J., and Sheppard, J. L. 1985. Seven-year longitudinal study of the early prediction of reading achievement. *Journal of Educational Psychology, 77*, 349—261.

Catts, H. W. 1986. Speech production/phonological deficits in reading-disordered children. *Journal of Learning Disabilities, 19*, 504—508.

Catts. H. W. 1989. Defining dyslexia as a developmental language disorder. *Annals of Dyslexia, 39*, 50—64.

Finucci, J. M., Gottfredson, L., and Childs, B. 1985. A follow-up study of dyslexic boys. *Annals of Dyslexia, 35*, 117—136.

Finucci, J. M., Guthrie, J. T., Childs, A. L., Abbey, H., and Childs, B. 1976. The genetics of specific reading disability. *Annals of Human Genetics, 40*, 1—23.

Fowler, A. E. 1988. Grammaticality judgments and reading skill in Grade 2. *Annals of Dyslexia, 38*, 73—94.

Gilger, J. W., Pennington, B. F., and DeFries, J. C. (in press). Risk for reading disability as a function of parental history in three family studies. *Reading and Writing: An Interdisciplinary Journal.*

Hallgren, B. 1950. Specific dyslexia ('congenital word blindness'): A clinical and genetic study. *Acta Psychiatrica et Neurologica, 65*, 1—287.

Hoien, T., Lundberg, I., Larsen, J. P., and Tonnesen, F. E. 1989. Profiles of reading-related skills in dyslexic families. *Reading and Writing, 1*, 381—392.

Jorm, A. F. and Share, D. L. 1983. Phonological recoding and reading acquisition. *Applied Psycholinguistics, 4*, 104—147.

Juel, C. 1988. Learning to read and write: A longitudinal study of 54 children through fourth grade. *Journal of Educational Psychology, 80*, 437—447.

Kagan, J. 1971. *Change and continuity in infancy*. New York: John Wiley and Sons.

Kerns, K. and Decker, S. N. 1985. Multifactorial assessment of reading disability: Identifying the best predictors. *Perceptual and Motor Skills, 60*, 747—753.

LaBuda, M. C. and DeFries, J. C. 1988. Cognitive abilities in children with reading disabilities. *Journal of Learning Disabilities, 21*, 562—566.

Lee, L. L. 1971. *Northwestern syntax screening test*. Evanston, IL: Northwestern University Press.

Liberman, I. Y. and Shankweiler, D. 1980. Speech, the alphabet and teaching to read. In L. B. Resnick and P. A. Weaver (eds.) *Theory and practice of early reading*. Hillsdale, NJ: Erlbaum.

Mann, V. A. 1984. Longitudinal prediction and prevention of early reading difficulty. *Annals of Dyslexia, 43*, 117—136.

Mann, V. A. and Ditunno, P. 1990. Phonological deficiencies: Effective predictors of future reading problems. *In* G. Pavlides (ed.), *Dyslexia: A neuropsychological and learning perspective*. NY: Wiley.

McCall, R. 1981. Nature-nurture and the two realms of development. *Child Development, 52*, 1—12.

Morrison, F. J. 1987. The nature of reading disability: Toward an integrative framework. *In* S. J. Ceci (ed.), *Handbook of cognitive, social, and neuropsychological aspects of learning disabilities*. Hillsdale, NJ: Erlbaum.

Richards, B. 1987. Type/token ratios: What do they really tell us? *Journal of Child Language, 14,* 201—209.
Rutter, M. and Yule, W. 1975. The concept of specific reading retardation. *Journal of Child Psychology and Psychiatry, 16,* 181—197.
Scarborough, H. S. 1984. Continuity between childhood dyslexia and adult reading. *British Journal of Psychology, 75,* 329—348.
Scarborough, H. S. 1989. Prediction of reading disability from familial and individual differences. *Journal of Educational Psychology, 81,* 101—108.
Scarborough, H. S. 1990a. Index of productive syntax. *Applied Psycholinguistics, 11,* 1—22.
Scarborough, H. S. 1990b. Very early language deficits in dyslexic children. *Child Development, 61*(6), 1728—1743.
Scarborough, H. S. (in press). Early syntactic development of dyslexic children. *Annals of Dyslexia.*
Scarborough, H. S. and Dobrich, W. 1990. Development of children with early language delay. *Journal of Speech and Hearing Research, 33,* 70—83.
Scarborough, H. S., Dobrich, W., and Hager, M. (in press). Preschool literacy experience and later reading achievement. *Journal of Learning Disabilities.*
Shankweiler, D. and Crain, S. 1986. Language mechanisms and reading disorder: A modular approach. *Cognition, 24,* 139—168.
Share, D. L., Jorm, A. F., Maclean, R., and Matthews, R. 1985. Sources of individual differences in reading acquisition. *Journal of Educational Psychology, 76,* 1309—1324.
Shaywitz, S. E., Shaywitz, B. A., Fletcher, J. M., and Escobar, M. D. 1990. Prevalence of reading disability in boys and girls. *Journal of the American Medical Association, 264,* 998—1002.
Stanovich, K. E. 1988. Explaining the differences between the dyslexic and the garden-variety poor reader: The phonological-core variable-difference model. *Journal of Learning Disabilities, 21,* 590—612.
Stanovich, K. E., Cunningham, A. E., and Cramer, B. B. 1984. Assessing phonological awareness in kindergarten children: Issues of task comparability. *Journal of Experimental Child Psychology, 38,* 175—190.
Teale, W. H. and Sulzby, E. (eds.) 1986. *Emergent literacy: Writing and reading.* Norwood, NJ: Ablex Press.
Vogler, G. P., DeFries, J. C., and Decker, S. N. 1985. Family history as an indicator of risk for reading disability. *Journal of Learning Disabilities, 18,* 419—421.
Wagner, R. K. and Torgesen, J. K. 1987. The nature of phonological processing and its causal role in the acquisition of reading skills. *Psychological Bulletin, 101,* 192—212.
Wells, G. 1986. Preschool literacy-related activities and success in school. *In* D. Olson, A. Hildyard, and N. Torrance (eds.), *Literacy, language and learning.* Cambridge: Cambridge University Press.
Woodcock, R. W. and Johnson, M. B. 1977. *Woodcock-Johnson psycho-educational battery.* Boston: Teaching Resources Corporation.
Zahalkova, M., Vrzal, V., and Kloboukova, E. 1972. Genetical investigations in dyslexia. *Journal of Medical Genetics, 9,* 48—52.

Confirmatory Factor Analysis of Word Recognition and Process Measures in the Colorado Reading Project

R. K. OLSON, J. J. GILLIS, J. P. RACK, J. C. DEFRIES and D. W. FULKER

Institute for Behavioral Genetics
University of Colorado
Boulder, Colorado

ABSTRACT: Measures of word recognition (REC) and two component skills, phonological coding (PHON) and orthographic coding (ORTH), were subjected to multivariate behavioral genetic analysis. Data were obtained from a sample of identical and fraternal twin pairs wherein at least one member of each pair was reading disabled (RD), and from a sample of twins wherein both members of each pair read in the normal range. Confirmatory factor analysis was used to fit the genetic, common environmental, and specific environmental covariance components for REC, PHON, and ORTH within the RD and normal simples. The resulting heritability estimates for REC, PHON, and ORTH were 0.59, 0.41, and 0.05 in the RD sample, and 0.35, 0.52, and 0.20 in the normal sample. After dropping the nonsignificant common environment parameters from the models, the genetic correlations between REC and PHON and between REC and ORTH were respectively 0.81 and 0.45 in the RD sample, and 0.68 and 0.45 in the normal sample. Differences between the genetic correlations were significant in the RD sample ($p < 0.005$), marginally significant in the normal sample ($p < 0.10$), and highly significant in the combined sample ($p < 0.001$), indicating that genetic influences on individual differences in REC are more strongly related to genetic variance in PHON than in ORTH. These results are consistent with previous demonstrations of substantial genetic covariance between the disabled group's deficits in REC and PHON, but not between REC and ORTH (Olson et al., 1989; Olson and Rack, 1990).

KEYWORDS: Word recognition, phonological, orthographic, genetics, dyslexia.

Primary goals of the Colorado Reading Project are to understand the genetic and environmental etiologies of reading disabilities and of individual differences in reading ability within the normal range. To achieve these goals, we compare the similarities of identical and fraternal twin pairs on a variety of reading and related process measures. If the degree of shared environment is approximately equal for the identical and fraternal pairs, greater similarity for the genetically identical twins provides evidence for genetic influence (Plomin, DeFries, and McClearn, 1990). In the present paper, confirmatory factor analysis of twin data is used to assess the etiology of variation in word recognition and two important com-

Reading and Writing: An Interdisciplinary Journal **3**: 235—248, 1991.
© 1991 *Kluwer Academic Publishers.*

ponent processes, as well as that of observed covariation among the three measures.

Comprehension of written text is a complex skill that depends on the integration of several component processes (Olson, Wise, Conners, and Rack, 1990). Verbal intelligence and word recognition have been identified as two major sources of independent variance in reading comprehension within both disabled and normal groups (Conners and Olson, 1990). Abilities such as oral vocabulary and general world knowledge, included under verbal intelligence, are needed to comprehend both spoken and written text, but skill in recognizing printed words is essential for fluent reading. Children with specific reading disability or dyslexia typically show deficits in word recognition that are inconsistent with their normal-range IQ and comprehension of spoken text.

Disabled readers' unique deficits in word recognition led us to examine two component processes that were initially based on the "dual route" model (Baron, 1977; Coltheart, 1978). In this model, words can be read by a slow "indirect" route that involves the sounding out of letters and letter clusters through the application of grapheme-phoneme correspondence rules. This is presumed to be the primary route for unfamiliar printed words and the most important route in the beginning stages of reading. A second rapid and "direct" or "visual" route, not dependent on phonological processes, is presumed to operate for the lexical identification of familiar printed words in skilled reading.

A number of recent criticisms have been directed toward the "dual route" model based on evidence that phonological processing is rapid and involuntary even for familiar printed words in skilled readers, and that the phonological decoding process may proceed by analogy with parts of familiar words rather than by grapheme-phoneme correspondence rules (Van Orden, Pennington, and Stone, 1990). Although this evidence suggests a primary role for phonological processes in both beginning and skilled reading, the homophonic nature of many English words requires the representation of specific orthographic patterns for lexical identification (e.g., there versus their; bear versus bare). In addition, there are many "exception" words that violate common phonological decoding rules (e.g., yacht). Therefore, both phonological coding and orthographic coding are necessary components in the recognition of printed English words. In the subsymbolic theory of Van Orden et al., word-specific orthographic knowledge is represented within the same processor that handles phonological coding, whereas in the dual process model, two independent processors are postulated.

Separate tasks were developed to assess skills in phonological coding and in the rapid identification of specific orthographic patterns (see Methods). Phonological coding required the rapid oral reading of a series of pronounceable nonwords (e.g., tegwop, framble). Orthographic coding required subjects to decide rapidly which of two homophonic letter strings was a real word (e.g., rane or rain). Phonological processes may be automatically elicited in the orthographic task, but they are not sufficient to decide on the correct response.

Previous analyses of disabled and normal readers' phonological and orthographic coding skills revealed that both accounted for independent variance in word recognition (Olson et al., 1990). However, the disabled readers' absolute levels of performance on the two tasks were different when compared to the performance of younger normal children at the same level of word recognition. The disabled readers' level of phonological coding was nearly a full standard deviation below that of the younger normal readers.

Our initial behavior-genetic analyses of word recognition, phonological coding, and orthographic coding focused on the etiology of the reading-disabled group's *deficits* (Olson, Wise, Conners, Rack, and Fulker, 1989). A twin sample was identified wherein at least one member was reading disabled (the proband). Then we compared the differential regression of the identical and fraternal cotwins' performance toward the mean of a normal control sample. If a deficit is completely heritable and there is no test error, genetically identical cotwins would be expected to show no regression to the population mean, while fraternal twins who share half their genes on average would regress half way toward the population mean. In the other extreme, if a deficit was due only to environmental influence, the identical and fraternal cotwins would show equal regression toward the population mean. Intermediate differences in identical and fraternal cotwin regression indicate the relative balance of genetic and environmental influences on the group deficit. A multiple regression procedure developed by DeFries and Fulker (1985) was used to estimate the degree of heritability (h^2_g) and shared environmental influences (c^2_g) for the probands' group deficit. Significant levels of heritability were found for deficits in word recognition and phonological coding, but not for orthographic coding (Olson et al., 1989). The most recent analyses with a substantially larger twin sample and more appropriate selection procedures yielded h^2_g estimates and standard errors of 0.44 ± 0.11 for word recognition, 0.75 ± 0.15 for phonological coding, and 0.31 ± 0.20 (n.s.) for orthographic coding (Olson and Rack, 1990). Estimates of shared environmental influences (c^2_g) were significant for deficits in word recognition (0.51 ± 0.11), and orthographic coding (0.48 ± 0.17), but not for phonological coding (0.12 ± 0.13, n.s.). Thus, the behavior-genetic analyses indicated significant genetic *and* shared environmental influences on group deficits in word recognition, significant genetic influences on group deficits in phonological coding, and significant shared environmental influences on group deficits in orthographic coding.

The above pattern of high h^2_g for phonological coding and low h^2_g for orthographic coding has also been suggested from data reported by Stevenson (this volume). Although his sample of reading disabled twins in London was comparatively small, Stevenson found significant estimates of heritability (h_g^2 = about 0.7) for deficits in judging whether two nonwords would sound the same when read aloud. Heritability estimates for deficits in accuracy for oral reading of nonwords were also moderately high (h_g^2 = about 0.5) but not significant in his small sample. Heritability estimates were generally negative and not significant for accuracy deficits in reading a list of exception words such as "yacht", which may predominantly tap subjects' orthographic coding skills. Thus, it is encouraging that our general pattern of higher heritability for phonological coding than for orthographic coding has been replicated in the London study. Contrary to the Colorado study, the London twins' deficits on a standardized word recognition measure (Schonell 1971) were not significantly heritable, although this may be due in part to the predominance of exception words in this test.

Now we turn to the main focus of the present paper, the heritability of individual differences in the normal range. Estimates of genetic and shared environmental influence on extreme group *deficits* (h_g^2 and c_g^2) do not necessarily reflect the pattern of genetic and shared environmental influences on individual differences *within* groups (h^2 and c^2), i.e., the etiology of extreme scores may differ from that of variation within the normal range. Recall that the statistical procedure for assessing the etiology of the probands' group deficit focuses on the differential regression of the MZ and DZ cotwins' group scores toward the normal population mean (DeFries and Fulker, 1985). This approach is quite different from the assessment of heritability for individual differences *within* the disabled and normal groups, which has been traditionally based on doubling the difference between intraclass correlations for identical and fraternal twins to obtain estimates of h^2 and c^2.

For an extreme (and unlikely) example of a contrast between h_g^2 and h^2 in a disabled twin sample, the MZ and DZ cotwin groups' means could regress equally to the population mean, indicating that the probands' *group* deficit is not due to heritable influences. (Such a result might be expected if one randomly chosen member of each twin pair was deprived of reading instruction while the other was given a good education.) However, the reading disabled probands may still vary in the severity of their reading deficit, and there may be differential covariance with the MZ and DZ cotwins' performance. It is theoretically possible that a much higher correlation for MZ than for DZ pairs could indicate high heritability for *within* group individual differences, in spite of low heritability for the probands' *group* deficit. Furthermore, it is theoretically plausible that the estimate for within-group heritability derived from the disabled twin sample is a valid index of heritability for individual differences in the normal range. In fact, we will show that estimates for h^2 within the disabled and normal twin groups are not significantly different.

DeFries and Fulker (1988) have formulated an extension of their regression procedure (DeFries and Fulker, 1985) that provides an assessment of h^2 and c^2 along with the significance of the difference between h^2 for individual differences in the population and h^2_g for the group deficit. (DeFries and Fulker noted that the power for this test is low and very large samples would be needed to reach acceptable levels of significance for all but the most extreme differences.) If significant, differences between h^2 and h^2_g would indicate a theoretically important difference in the relative influence of genetic and environmental factors on individual variation in the population versus the extreme-group deficits of disabled readers. However, such differences would not necessarily indicate differences in the underlying genetic mechanism. For example, it would be possible that the same gene or genes are responsible for both normal and extremely deviant variation in reading, but in the deviant cases there is a uniquely potent environmental effect, leading to a lower h^2_g.

In the present paper, we employ confirmatory factor analyses of twin data to assess genetic and shared environmental influences on individual differences within the normal range. This approach facilitates estimates of h^2 and c^2 for word recognition and the component coding skills, as well as estimates of the genetic correlations among the three measures. A genetic correlation provides a measure of the extent to which individual differences in two characters are due to the same genetic influences (Plomin et al., 1990). Through confirmatory factor analysis we will directly assess the degree to which genetic variance in phonological coding and orthographic coding is correlated with genetic variance in word recognition. In addition, we will determine whether the genetic correlations with word recognition are significantly different for phonological and orthographic coding. Data from the disabled twin group, the normal twin group, and the combined group will be subjected to separate analyses.

METHODS

Subjects

Two groups of twins between 7 and 20 years of age were ascertained from school records in 27 Colorado districts. In the disabled group, at least one member of each pair had a positive history of reading problems in their school records, and when tested in the laboratory on the word recognition, reading comprehension and spelling subtests of the Peabody Individual Achievement Test (PIAT; Dunn and Markwardt, 1970), they were below a discriminant function score previously established to discriminate independent samples of 140 disabled and 140 normal readers (DeFries, 1985). In the normal comparison group, there was no evidence in the school records for reading problems in either twin and both twins scored above the critical discriminant function score. Additional inclusionary criteria for twins in both groups were a score of at least 90 on the Wechsler (1974) Verbal or Performance subscales, no evidence of neurological problems such as seizures, no uncorrected visual acuity or auditory deficits, and English was the primary language spoken in the home. The disabled group contained 86 identical or monozygotic (MZ) twin pairs and 73 same-sex fraternal or dizygotic (DZ) pairs. The normal group contained 92 MZ pairs and 59 same-sex DZ pairs. The twins' zygosity was determined using selected items from the Nichols and Bilbro (1966) zygosity questionnaire which has a reported accuracy of 95%.

Measures

A battery of reading and related cognitive measures, including the PIAT and Wechsler tests, was administered to the twins in DeFries' laboratory at the Institute for Behavior Genetics. Experimental measures of reading and related processes, including phonological and orthographic coding, were administered in a second session at Olson's laboratory in the Department of Psychology. Because the present analyses focus on PIAT word recognition, phonological coding, and orthographic coding, only these measures are described here. More complete descriptions are given in Olson et al. (1990).

PIAT Word Recognition (REC) (Dunn and Markwart, 1970). This standardized test consists of a series of 66 unrelated words placed in rows across several pages in order of increasing difficulty. Subjects were asked to read the words across the rows until they made five errors on the last seven items. The test-retest reliability is reported to be 0.89 across grade levels 1—12. Most of the words are regularly spelled and the subjects had unlimited time to reach each word.

Phonological Coding (PHON). This experimental task required subjects to read a block of 45 one-syllable nonwords (e.g., ter, calch, doun), followed by a block of 40 two-syllable nonwords (e.g., tegwop, stalder, framble), as quickly and accurately as possible when the nonwords appeared individually on a computer screen. Oral responses were timed with a voice key and were tape recorded for later scoring of percent correct. A response was considered correct if it followed grapheme-phoneme correspondence rules (tive pronounced to rhyme with hive), or by analogy to an orthographically similar word (tive pronounced to rhyme with give). *Z* scores for percent correct and mean response time on correct trials were combined for each block, and a final score was derived by adding the combined z scores for the two blocks.

Orthographic Coding (ORTH). This experimental task required subjects to designate the word in word-pseudohomophone pairs as quickly as possible by pushing a right or left button after the pairs were presented on the computer monitor. The stimuli in each pair ranged from relatively short and frequent words (e.g., room-rume, rane-rain, sleep-sleap) in the first block of 40 trials to longer and less frequent words (e.g., sammon-salmon, explaine-explain) in the second block of 40 trials. Subjects were shown their response time in msec. after correct responses, and were shown the word "error" after incorrect responses. Z scores for percent correct and response time on correct trials were combined for each block, and a final score was derived by adding the combined z scores for the two blocks.

ANALYSES AND RESULTS

The twins' scores on each of the above measures were adjusted for their linear relation to age and standardized based on the mean and standard deviation in the normal sample. Although the mean of the disabled sample was therefore substantially lower, the variance was similar to that of the normal sample, thus reflecting a wide range of reading deficit.

In order to estimate genetic variances and covariances, the age-adjusted standardized scores for REC, PHON, and ORTH were subjected to multivariate behavioral genetic analysis (Fulker, Baker, and Bock, 1983; DeFries and Fulker, 1986; Heath, Neale, Hewitt, Eaves, and Fulker, 1989). Observed MZ and DZ cross-covariance matrices were fit to a simple factor model that included one common factor and three specific variances. The factor loadings in the full model were estimated from the phenotypic correlations using confirmatory factor analysis. An expected covariance matrix, [E], was compared to the observed phenotypic covariance matrix, [P], using the following log-likelihood function:

$$F = N[\log_e(\mathrm{DET}[E]/\mathrm{DET}[P]) + \mathrm{tr}([P]\,[E]^{-1}) - k],$$

where N is the degrees of freedom for subjects, and k is the number of variables. The function was minimized using the MINUIT optimization package (CERN, 1977). The change in chi-square values for reduced models as compared to the full model was used to test the significance of factors in a given model.

Observed covariances between the REC, PHON, and ORTH variables were partitioned into genetic, common environmental, and specific environmental components as follows:

$$[P] = [G] + [C] + [S],$$

where [P] is the phenotypic variance/covariance matrix, and [G], [C], and [S] are the additive genetic, common environmental, and specific environmental (including measurement error) component matricies, respectively. The genetic and environmental covariances were assumed to be uncorrelated.

Confirmatory factor analyses were first performed separately for the reading disabled and normal groups (results of these analyses were previously summarized in an abstract by Gillis, DeFries, Olson, and Rack, 1990). The phenotypic correlations for REC, PHON, and ORTH in the disabled and normal groups are presented in Table 1. In both groups, the correlation between REC and PHON is higher than that between REC and ORTH, although the difference is significant ($p < 0.025$) in only the disabled group. This result is partly due to the lower reliability of the forced-choice ORTH task, and partly due to the fact that most words in the REC measure were phonologically regular and could be phonologically decoded without memory for their specific orthographic patterns. Correlations were higher between ORTH and a timed experimental word recognition measure that included about half regular and half irregular words (Olson et al., 1990).

The full model yielded the estimates of heritability (h^2) and shared environment (c^2) presented in Table 2. It can be seen that the heritability estimates for REC and PHON range from 0.35 to 0.59 across the disabled and control groups, but the heritability for ORTH is only 0.05 in the disabled group and 0.20 in the control group. Estimates of shared environment are low except for ORTH (0.47) in the disabled group. The pattern of higher heritability for REC and PHON compared to ORTH is

Table 1. Phenotypic correlations among Word Recognition (REC), Phonological Coding (PHON), and Orthographic Coding (ORTH) measures

	Reading disabled				Controls		
	REC	*PHON*	*ORTH*		*REC*	*PHON*	*ORTH*
REC	1.00	0.65	0.30	REC	1.00	0.55	0.33
PHON		1.00	0.41	PHON		1.00	0.34
ORTH			1.00	ORTH			1.00

$N_{MZ} = 86$ pairs
$N_{DZ} = 73$ pairs

$N_{MZ} = 92$ pairs
$N_{DZ} = 59$ pairs

Table 2. Heritability (h^2) and Shared Environment (c^2) for Word Recognition (REC), Phonological Coding (PHON), and Orthographic Coding (ORTH)[a]

Reading disabled				Controls			
	h^2	c^2	$(h^2)^b$		h^2	c^2	$(h^2)^b$
REC	0.59	0.00	0.58	REC	0.35	0.24	0.60
PHON	0.41	0.07	0.49	PHON	0.52	0.01	0.53
ORTH	0.05	0.47	0.52	ORTH	0.20	0.20	0.40

[a] h^2 and c^2 estimates are for the full model.
[b] (h^2) estimates are based on dropping c^2 from the model.

consistent with the results of the Olson et al. (1989) and Olson and Rack (1990) analyses for the heritability of the disabled groups' deficits (h_g^2) on these measures.

Table 3 summarizes the results of fitting alternative multivariate models of genetic and shared environmental influence to data for the three variables in the two samples. Significant changes in chi-square and deterioration of model fit occurred when genetic factors [G] were dropped for both the reading disabled and control groups. In contrast, shared environmental factors [C] could be dropped in both groups without a significant change in chi-square. Therefore, shared environment was dropped from the model to facilitate a more powerful test of the genetic correlations between the variables. The resulting correlations are presented in Table 4. In both groups, the genetic correlation between REC and PHON is greater than that between REC and ORTH. Constraining these correlations to be equal in the model led to a highly significant deterioration of fit in the disabled group ($\chi^2 = 11.36$, df = 1, $p < 0.005$), and a marginally significant deterioration of fit in the control group ($\chi^2 = 3.36$, df = 1, $p < 0.10$).

The pattern of genetic correlations was similar in the disabled and

Table 3. Model fitting results

			Reading disabled			Controls		
Model	df	Δ df	χ^2	$\Delta\chi^2$	p	χ^2	$\Delta\chi^2$	p
Full Model	24		54.14		<0.025	72.64		<0.005
Drop [G]	30	6	73.61	19.47	<0.005	87.38	14.74	<0.025
Drop [C]	30	6	63.72	9.58	>0.10	77.51	4.87	>0.50
Drop [C] and [G]	36	12	137.75	83.61	<0.005	160.61	87.97	<0.005

Table 4. Genetic correlations among Word Recognition (REC), Phonological Coding (PHON), and Orthographic Coding (ORTH) measures

Reading disabled				Controls			
	REC	*PHON*	*ORTH*		*REC*	*PHON*	*ORTH*
REC	1.00	0.81	0.45	REC	1.00	0.68	0.45
PHON		1.00	0.56	PHON		1.00	0.52
ORTH			1.00	ORTH			1.00

control samples, as indicated by the test of homogeneity presented in Table 5. Therefore, the groups were combined for a final analysis. The genetic correlations were 0.75 for REC and PHON, 0.42 for REC and ORTH, and 0.56 for PHON and ORTH. Constraining the genetic correlations between REC and PHON (r_{g12}) and between REC an ORTH (r_{g13}) to be equal in the model yielded a highly significant deterioration in fit ($\chi^2 = 14.78, df = 1, p < 0.001$).

It should be emphasized that it was necessary to drop shared environment from the model to obtain significant contrasts between genetic correlations. This is partly due to the very low heritabilities for ORTH in the full model (see Table 2), which resulted in highly unstable estimates of genetic correlations between REC and ORTH. For example, when shared environment was included in the model for the disabled group, the genetic correlation between REC and ORTH was estimated to be 1.00, but with a standard error of 0.63! The primary effect of dropping shared environment was to increase the heritability estimate for ORTH from 0.05 in the

Table 5. Model fitting results from the combined reading disabled and control twin samples

	Combined reading disabled and control sample				
Model	df	χ^2	Δ df	$\Delta\chi^2$	p
Estimate [G] and [S]: RD	30	63.72			
Estimate [G] and [S]: Controls	30	77.51			
Estimate [G] and [S]: Combined	72	150.57			
Homogeneity			12	9.34	>0.50
Constrain r_{g12}[a] = r_{g13}[b]	73	165.35			
Difference			1	14.78	<0.001

[a] Genetic correlation between REC and PHON.
[b] Genetic correlation between REC and ORTH.

full model for disabled readers to 0.52 for the more parsimonious model. With this constraint, the genetic correlation between REC and ORTH was 0.45 with a standard error of 0.09, enabling a significant contrast with the much higher genetic correlation of 0.81 ± 0.14 between REC and PHON. Nevertheless, results of fitting both models indicate that the genetic *covariance* between ORTH and REC is substantially lower than that between PHON and REC.

DISCUSSION

The confirmatory factor analyses showed remarkable agreement in the results for the disabled and normal groups, even though the disabled group was highly selected. There was a similar degree of genetic influence on within group individual differences in word recognition and phonological coding. This result suggests that genetic factors operate in a similar way on individual differences in word recognition and phonological coding within the normal range and within the low tail of the distribution, although it is possible that the specific genes influencing individual differences could vary across the range of ability (Pennington, 1989).

Another striking result was the absence of significant shared environment influences, as these could be dropped from the model without a significant deterioration in fit. Therefore, genetic and non-shared environmental factors were the predominant etiological basis for within-group individual differences in word recognition and phonological coding. However, the results for orthographic coding were not as clear, particularly in the disabled group. Although the c^2 estimate of 0.47 for orthographic coding was not statistically significant in our small sample, it suggests the strong possibility of shared environmental influences. Such a result would be consistent with Olson and Rack's (1990) previous c_g^2 estimates for the group deficit in orthographic coding to be discussed later.

The most significant results from the confirmatory factor analyses were the contrasts in genetic correlations between word recognition and the two coding measures. Genetic influences on word recognition and phonological coding are highly correlated in both groups, and these correlations are significantly higher than those for word recognition and orthographic coding.

The above results are consistent with differences in genetic *covariance* previously reported between the disabled group's deficits in word recognition, phonological coding, and orthographic coding (Olson et al., 1989; Olson and Rack, 1990). (A genetic correlation is a function of both the genetic covariance between the two variables *and* of their heritabilities. Thus, even if the covariance between genetic influences on two variables is low, the genetic correlation could be high if one or both variables has a low heritability.) The most recent analyses by Olson and Rack (1990) yielded evidence for significant genetic covariance ("bivariate h_g^2"), but no significant environmental covariance, between probands' deficits in word recognition and cotwins' phonological coding (h_g^2 = 0.73 ± 0.17; c_g^2 = 0.22 ± 0.14). In contrast, for word recognition and orthographic coding, there was no significant genetic covariance, but shared environmental covariance was significant (h_g^2 = 0.32 ± 0.25, n.s.; c_g^2 = 0.60 ± 0.20).

Olson and Rack's (1990) estimate of h_g^2 = 0.75 ± 0.15 for the group deficit in phonological coding is somewhat higher than the h^2 estimates for within-group individual differences presented in Table 2. Our twin sample is still too small for the contrast between h_g^2 and h^2 to be statistically significant in DeFries and Fulker's (1988) augmented model, but the current trend suggests a stronger genetic influence on disabled readers' deficits in phonological coding than on individual differences in phonological coding within the normal range.

The h^2 and h_g^2 estimates for word recognition were similar at about 0.5, but the absence of c^2 (0.00) for individual differences within the disabled group contrasts sharply with our most recent estimate of shared environment for the disabled group's deficit in word recognition (c_g^2 = 0.51 ± 0.11). These results suggest that shared environmental influences may be an important cause of the group deficit in word recognition, but not of individual differences within the group.

Shared environment was also significant for group deficits in orthographic coding (c_g^2 = 0.48 ± 0.17), and there was substantial shared environmental covariance for probands' deficits in word recognition and cotwins' orthographic coding (c_g^2 = 0.60 ± 0.20) (Olson and Rack, 1990). In agreement with Stanovich and West (1989), we have argued that exposure to print is an important factor in the development of orthographic skills in word recognition, and print exposure is likely to be influenced by the twins' shared environment (Olson et al., 1990). Consistent with this view, orthographic coding manifested comparable levels of c^2 (0.47) and c_g^2 (0.48) for the disabled group. We should add a caveat that just as similar estimates of h^2 and h_g^2 do not necessarily imply the same specific genetic mechanism, it is theoretically possible that the specific shared environmental influences are different, even if estimates of c^2 and c_g^2 are similar.

In contrast to word recognition and orthographic coding, estimates of the proportion of variance due to shared environmental influences for phonological coding have *never* been significant in either the present analyses of within-group differences or in previous analyses of the group deficit. Genetic factors and non-shared environment are consistently the predominant causes of variance in phonological coding, and most of the heritable variance in word recognition is shared with heritable variance in phonological coding. Stanovich (1988) has emphasized the central role of phonological coding for reading disabilities in his "phonological-core variable-difference model". Results of the present study suggest that it is also central to the eitology of individual differences within the normal range.

ACKNOWLEDGMENTS

This work was supported in part by program project and center grants from the NICHD (HD-11681 and HD-27802). This report was prepared while J. Gillis was supported by NIMH training grant MH-16880. The invaluable contributions of staff members of the many Colorado school districts that participate in our research, and of the twins and their families, are gratefully acknowledged.

REFERENCES

Baron, J. 1977. Mechanisms for pronouncing printed words: use and acquisition. In D. Laberge and S. J. Samuels (Eds.), *Basic processes in reading: perception and comprehension*. Hillsdale, NJ. Erlbaum.

Cern. 1977. MINUIT: A system for Function Minimization and Analysis of Parameter Errors and Correlations, CERN, Geneva, Switzerland.

Coltheart, M. 1978. Lexical access in simple reading tasks. In G. Underwood (Ed.), *Strategies of information processing*. London: Academic Press.

Conners, F. and Olson, R. K. 1990. Reading comprehension in dyslexic and normal readers: A component-skills analysis. In D. A. Balota, G. B. Flores d'Arcais, and K. Rayner (Eds.), *Comprehension processes in reading* (pp. 557—579). Hillsdale, NJ: Erlbaum.

DeFries, J. C. 1985. Colorado reading project. In D. B. Gray and J. F. Kavanagh (Eds.), *Biobehavioral measures of dyslexia* (pp. 107—122). Parkton, MD: York Press.

DeFries, J. C. and Fulker, D. W. 1986. Multivariate behavioral genetics and development: An overview. *Behavior Genetics, 16*, 1—10.

DeFries, J. C. and Fulker, D. W. 1985. Multiple regression analysis of twin data. *Behavior Genetics, 15*, 467—473.

DeFries, J. C. and Fulker, D. W. 1988. Multiple regression analysis of twin data: Etiology of deviant scores versus individual differences. *Acta Geneticae Medicae et Gemellologiae: Twin Research, 37*, 205—216.

Dunn, L. M. and Markwardt, F. C. 1970. *Examiner's manual: Peabody Individual Achievement Test*, Circle Pines, MN: American Guidance Service.

Fulker, D. W., Baker, L. A. and Bock, R. D. 1983. Estimating components of covariation using LISREL. *Data Analysis, 1*, 5—8.

Gillis, J. J., DeFries, J. C., Olson, R. K. and Rack, J. P. 1990. Confirmatory factor analysis of reading performance and process measures in the Colorado Reading Project. *Behavior Genetics, 20* 721 (Abstract).

Heath, A. C., Neale. M. C., Hewitt, J. K., Eaves, L. J. and Fulker, D. W. 1989. Testing structural equation models for twin data using LISREL. *Behavior Genetics, 19*, 9—35.

Nichols, R. C. and Bilbro, W. C. 1966. The diagnosis of twin zygosity. *Acta Genetica, 16,* 265—275.

Olson, R. K. and Rack, J. P. 1990. *Genetic and environmental influences on component reading and language skills.* Paper presented at the XVI International Rodin Remediation Scientific Conference on Genetic and Neurological Influences in Dyslexia, Boulder, Colorado, September 19—21, 1990.

Olson, R. K., Wise, B., Conners, F. and Rack, J. 1990. Organization, heritability, and remediation of component word recognition and language skills in disabled readers. In T. H. Carr and B. A. Levy (Eds.), *Reading and its development: Component skills approaches* (pp. 261—322). New York: Academic Press.

Olson, R. K., Wise, B., Conners, F., Rack, J. and Fulker, D. 1989. Specific deficits in component reading and language skills: Genetic and environmental influences. *Journal of Learning Disabilities, 22,* 339—348.

Plomin, R., DeFries, J. C. and McClearn, G. E. 1990. *Behavioral Genetics: A Primer.* New York: W. H. Freeman and Company.

Pennington, B. F. 1989. Using genetics to understand dyslexia. *Annals of Dyslexia, 39,* 81—93.

Schonell, F. J. 1971. *Reading and Spelling Tests: Handbook of Instructions.* Edinburgh: Oliver and Boyd.

Stanovich, K. E. 1988. Explaining the differences between the dyslexic and the garden-variety poor reader: the phonological-core variable-difference model. *Journal of Learning Disabilities, 21,* 590—612.

Stanovich, K. E. and West, R. F. 1989. Exposure to print and orthographic processing. *Reading Research Quarterly, 24,* 402—433.

Stevenson, J. (in press). Which aspects of processing text mediate genetic effects? *Reading and Writing: An Interdisciplinary Journal.*

Van Orden, G. C., Pennington, B. F. and Stone, G. O. 1990. Word identification in reading and the promise of subsymbolic psycholinguistics. *Psychological Review, 97,* 488—522.

Wechsler, D. 1974. *Examiner's manual: Wechsler Intelligence Scale for Children-Revised.* New York: The Psychological Corporation.

Which Aspects of Processing Text Mediate Genetic Effects?

JIM STEVENSON

Department of Psychology
University of Surrey
Guildford, England

ABSTRACT. Genetic influences on reading are investigated in a sample of 285, 13 year old twins. Using a multiple regression procedure, the heritability of disability (h_g^2) for Reading Recognition was found to be non-significant. However the h_g^2 for spelling disability was found to be 0.58 ($P < 0.05$), after controlling for individual differences in IQ. The twins in this study were an unselected sample from the general population. Therefore it was possible to estimate h_g^2 for differing degrees of severity of disability. These analyses showed that for spelling but not for Reading Recognition or Reading Composite, there were substantial genetic contributions to all levels of disability. For indices of Orthographic Coding there were no significant values of h_g^2. In contrast measures of Phonological Coding and Homophone Recognition have consistently high values of h_g^2. More detailed analyses suggested that there were possibly *two* independent aspects of phonological ability, each influenced by genetic factors.

KEYWORDS: genetic, reading, spelling, phonological ability, twin study

Despite some doubts expressed over their applicability (Hay et al., 1984), the clearest specific tests of genetic aetiology of reading disability have been twin studies. A number of early twin studies (e.g. Bakwin, 1973; Zerbin-Rudin, 1967) were undertaken but suffered from a number of methodological problems that make the results of historical interest only (see Stevenson et al., 1987 for a review). Apart from the somewhat smaller study of Harris (1986) the two largest recent twin studies have been the Colorado Reading Study (DeFries, Fulker and LaBuda, 1987, DeFries, 1988) and that carried out in London (Stevenson, Graham, Fredman and McLoughlin, 1987; Fredman and Stevenson, 1988; Stevenson and Fredman, 1990).

The Colorado research has found higher MZ than DZ concordance rates, which were consistent with higher heritability for reading per se. The concordance rates in the London study indicated that the effects of genetic influences, once general intelligence was controlled by regression, were greatest for spelling ability. Aspects of reading ability showed only modest and non-significant heritabilities.

Reading and Writing: An Interdisciplinary Journal 3: 249–269, 1991.
© 1991 *Kluwer Academic Publishers.*

MULTIPLE REGRESSION ANALYSIS OF TWIN DATA

There are now a number of more appropriate methods of treating such twin data that go beyond comparisons of concordance rates. The significance of the emergence of multiple regression analysis of twin data has been its power to detect genetic influences based upon selected samples of twins where at least one member of the pair is a proband. The technique is based on the equation:

$$C = B_1P + B_2R + A \ldots [1]$$

where C is the cotwin's predicted score, P is the proband's score, R is the coefficient of relationship and A is a constant (DeFries, Fulker and LaBuda, 1987).

THE LONDON TWIN READING STUDY

The twins in the present sample were obtained via birth records from hospitals in 5 London boroughs and from a search of the registers of schools in the Inner London Area. Although there were some refusals to co-operate with the study, the sample has proved to share very similar characteristics to non-twin children living in the same area (Graham and Stevenson, 1985; Stevenson, Graham, Fredman and McLoughlin, 1987). It is therefore a representative sample of twin children, who were tested on a number of tests including the Neale Analysis of Reading Ability (Neale, 1967), the Schonell Single Word Reading and Spelling Tests (Schonell and Schonell, 1960) and the Wechsler Intelligence Scale for Children-Revised (Wechsler, 1974). The children were also given a number of other single word reading tasks (Coltheart, 1981). These were designed to assess aspects of Phonological and Orthographic Coding (see Fredman and Stevenson, 1988 for full details). Phonological Coding was tested by the child reading aloud non-words (e.g. bue, owt, woz). These could only be read by some non-lexical process i.e. either using grapheme-phoneme correspondences or by analogy with parts of words. Orthographic Coding was tested using irregular or exception words aloud (e.g. answer, break, yacht, gross). During neither of these tasks were the subjects put under any time constraint; they were able to read the material aloud at their own preferred rate. It would have been valuable to have had a more extensive assessment of both phonological and orthographic ability. In particular it would have been preferable if the test of non-word reading had used more complex letter strings than the trigraphs used. More importantly the reading of irregular or exception words is only a partial test of orthographic ability. The addition of a task such as that adopted by Olson et al. (1989) using word identification in pseudo-homophone pairs would have been advantageous.

A further set of tasks required the child to judge whether pairs of letter strings sounded the same or different. These did not have to be read aloud, indeed the child was asked to do the task silently. The material included three tasks that comprised in turn pairs of non-words, regular and irregular words where words or letter strings that sounded the same had to be identified. The pairs that sounded the same were true homophones (e.g. "higher" and "hire"). The results were similar for all types of reading material and therefore an aggregated measure was obtained from the sum of child's z scores on these three tasks and was called Homophone Recognition.

The Colorado Reading Study results usually include an analysis of a summary score derived from a discriminant analysis using the pooled cognitive measures to predict group membership for an independent sample of reading disabled non-twin subjects and controls. In order to generate a similar type of composite measure the Neale Analysis of Reading Ability Accuracy and Comprehension Scores and the Schonell Single Word Reading and Spelling scores for all twins were subjected to a principal component analysis. The results are summarised in Table 1. A single factor solution was produced which explained 85.9% of the variance and the twin's scores on this factor were calculated (Reading Composite).

DATA ANALYSIS

For each of the reading and spelling measures the following data analysis was undertaken based upon the procedures for multiple regression analysis of twin data (DeFries and Fulker, 1985, 1988). The opposite-sex DZ twin pairs were excluded. The mean scores for MZ and DZ pairs were compared using a t-test. If there were significant differences between the zygosity groups the scores were converted to deviation scores from the zygosity group mean and then divided by the zygosity group standard deviation. If there was not a significant difference between zygosity group means, the scores were expressed as deviations from the mean of pooled MZ and DZ scores and then divided by the standard deviation of these pooled scores. The "deviant" cases (probands) were identified by using a criterion of scoring more than a given number of standard deviations below the total group mean. Where both members of a twin pair met the criterion for proband they were both entered into the analysis as proband and cotwin in turn. This form of "double entry" analysis is considered the most appropriate with truncate selection (Thompson and Thompson,

Table 1. Factor analysis of main reading variables used to derive Reading Composite measure

	Factor Loadings	Communality
Neale Accuracy	0.970	0.941
Neale Comprehension	0.840	0.705
Schonell Spelling	0.927	0.858
Schonell Reading	0.965	0.932
Eigen value	3.436	
% variance explained	85.9%	

Correlation of factor score with Full Scale WISC-R IQ $r = 0.71$
Regression on Full Scale IQ = (0.046 × WISC-R IQ) − 4.58

1986). It requires a correction to be made to the standard errors obtained from the multiple regression analysis of the following form:

$$\text{Corrected Standard Error} = \text{Obtained Standard Error} \times \sqrt{(N_D - K - 1)/(N_S - K - 1)} \ldots [2]$$

N_D = number of double entry probands
N_S = number of single entry probands
K = number of coefficients in regression equation

For each zygosity separately each child's score was divided by the difference between the mean for the probands of that zygosity and the total group mean. The final stage of the data analysis was to derive the regression coefficients in equation [1].

THE VALUE OF TOTAL TWIN SAMPLE

There was no scope for testing the hypothesis of age related effects within the London twin sample since all the twins were tested within a few months of their thirteenth birthdays. However there are a number of features of the data set that are of particular value especially when allied to multiple regression analysis. The twins were an unselected sample of the twins living in the area and therefore the effects of defining deviant group membership in alternative ways can be investigated. In this paper, findings will be presented that use this feature of the study to investigate:

1. whether the London and Colorado samples produce congruent values for h_g^2 for similar definitions of reading disability.
2. whether h_g^2 changes with severity of reading disability.

3. whether h_g^2 changes with severity of disability for components of the reading process.
4. which aspects of phonological ability are influenced by genetic factors.

REPLICATION OF SOME OF THE RECENT FINDINGS ON GENETIC INFLUENCES ON READING PROCESS MEASURES

It is of interest to establish whether the data from the London twin study replicates the findings being produced by the Colorado group (Olson et al., 1989, Olson and Rack, 1990). An overview of their findings has been given in Table 2 and as far as possible parallel findings from the London study are given in the top half of Table 3. It should be noted that as with previous findings from the studies the Colorado results show a higher heritability for word recognition than London (see also Olson et al., 1991 for further details of the findings from the Colorado Reading Project).

There are some important differences in the ways the analyses for the two studies were conducted. First, the findings in Olson et al. (1989) are based upon single entry regression analyses whereas those in the Olson and Rack (1990) and the London study reported here are based upon double entry regression analyses. As was mentioned above, the double entry method is considered to be more appropriate for the method of proband selection used in these twin studies. Second the results given in Olson et al. (1989) were based upon proband defined as being low scoring on word recognition as well as showing phonological or orthographic

Table 2. Summary of the values for the heritability of disability (h_g^2) for components of reading ability

Measure	Age range	N_{mz} pairs	N_{dz} pairs	h_g^2	Standard error
Olson et al. (1989)					
Word recognition	7:7–20:4	64	53	0.40^{+++}	$0.11^{\$}$
WR adjusted by intelligence		—	—	0.37^{++}	$0.13^{\$}$
Phonological coding		—	—	0.46^{++}	0.15
Orthographic coding		—	—	0.28	0.17
Olson and Rack (1990)					
Word recognition	mean 12.5	95	106	0.46^{+}	0.13
Phonological coding		98	88	0.65^{+}	0.16
Orthographic coding		68	65	0.23	0.23

$^{\$}$ converted from 95% CI
$^{+}$ $P < 0.05$, $^{++}$ $P < 0.01$, $^{+++}$ $P < 0.001$

Table 3. Values for deviant group heritability (h_g^2) for groups defined by being < −1.00 standard deviation below population mean for each respective dimension

Measure	Age range	N_{mz} pairs	N_{dz}	h_g^2	Standard error
Basic reading scores					
Word recognition single words	13:0—13:6	23	42	0.03	0.37
Reading composite		19	46	0.21	0.38
Spelling		19	43	0.47	0.33
Phonological coding		27	36	0.41	0.39
Orthographic coding		6	30	−0.91	0.53
IQ adjusted					
Word recognition single words		20	38	0.03	0.37
Reading composite		20	38	0.01	0.40
Spelling		30	38	0.58^{+}	0.34
Phonological coding				0.36	0.39
Orthographic coding				−0.68	0.56

deficits. These are not pure estimates of h_g^2 for phonological and orthographic coding. The estimates presented by Olson and Rack (1990) are more strictly replicates of those obtained from the London data. In both cases double entry methods were used and probands were identified simply by being low scorers on the phonological or orthographic coding measures alone. There are some parallels between the London and Colorado studies especially in finding higher h_g^2 for Phonological Coding than for Orthographic Coding. This difference is also reflected in the heritability of individual differences (h^2) for these measures in the London study. Stevenson (in press) obtained a value of h^2 for Phonological Coding of 0.50 and of 0.04 for Orthographic Coding.

It is important to note here that although the procedures for measuring Phonological Coding were very similar in the two studies (i.e. reading aloud of one or two syllable pronounceable non-words), the tests of Orthographic Coding were different. In the London study this was indexed by the child reading aloud irregular words i.e. that do not conform to normal spelling rules. In Colorado the child had to identify the word in a non-word/word homophone pair. In both cases it is argued that the task requires the child to read using whole word or lexical processes and therefore is sensitive to Orthographic Coding ability.

The Colorado and London twin studies use different methods to control for the relationship between intelligence and reading (Siegel, 1989). The Colorado sample was restricted to those cases with IQs above 90. There were no sample selection restrictions made in the London study. Intelligence was controlled by multiple regression before h_g^2 analyses were undertaken. In Table 3 and succeeding tables results are presented both for measures without IQ control and for the residual scores after regression onto IQ. There is a moderate h^2 for intelligence from twins reared together of about 0.52 (see Plomin and Loehlin, 1989 for a discussion of variations from this estimate). Even given a conservative estimate of the correlation between IQ and reading of 0.4 (Torgesen, 1989), it can always be argued that genetic analyses applied to raw reading scores might only be sensitive to genetic effects on that part of variance in reading that is a reflection of IQ differences between children. In this sense estimates of h_g^2 obtained from reading score residuals after regression onto IQ provide an index of more specific genetic effects related to reading. As can be seen in the lower half of Table 3 the effect of using an IQ control is to enhance the value of h_g^2 for spelling which then reaches significance ($P < 0.05$). These findings run counter to the position of Siegel (1989) who suggested that IQ control was unnecessary when defining and investigating reading disabilities.

There were a number of findings concerning the relationship between IQ, word recognition and other reading scores produced by Olson et al. (1989). Within the reading disabled group they report $r = 0.35$ between word recognition and IQ. The London twins produce $r = 0.26$ for these measures. The level of reading disability was estimated to be −2.4 standard deviations in Colorado for the group below −1 S. D. The London twin probands were less deviant. Their mean word recognition scores were −1.8 standard deviations below the total sample mean. The Colorado measures of Phonological and Orthographic Coding were only modestly correlated within the reading disabled group ($r = 0.25$). The result for London was similar ($r = 0.32$). There was a difference however in the correlations between Phonological and Orthographic Coding and Word Recognition within the reading disabled group. In London the correlations were 0.40 and 0.86, whilst in Colorado they were 0.69 and 0.40. The higher correlations between Orthographic Coding and Word Recognition in the London sample can be explained by the high frequency of exception words in the Schonell Graded Word Reading Test (used as the measure of Word Recognition for the London sample).

MULTIPLE REGRESSION ANALYSES TO TEST h_g^2 FOR DEGREES OF READING DISABILITY

The following analyses attempt to establish whether genetic effects on reading processes show a substantial change in the mix of causal factors as more extreme definitions of disability are identified. This would be reflected in a varying estimate for h_g^2 across the range. This can be tested in a sample such as that from London, by estimating h_g^2 using differing degrees of severity to identify probands.

The results relevant to this issue have been presented in a common format in Tables 4 to 8. In each case a multiple regression analysis has been undertaken using an increasingly severe definition of disability in terms of standard deviation units relative to the sample mean. It should be noted that Phonological and Orthographic Coding are error scores and therefore scores above the mean indicate disability.

It is important to recognise a number of limitations on this analysis. Firstly there were insufficient pairs to test for differences between h^2 and h_g^2 using the augmented model (DeFries and Fulker, 1985). Secondly, the numbers of probands in the more extreme groups are often small. The standard errors of B_2 (h_g^2) are therefore large and it is therefore difficult to establish whether the B_2 are significantly greater than zero. However the results are given applying one-tailed tests to these regression coefficients. Thirdly, demonstrating a sustained value for h_g^2 across a range of disabilities does not necessarily imply that the same genetic or the same environmental processes are acting. Identical values of h_g^2 could be produced by quite different genetic and environmental factors; it is only an index of their net effects.

From the basic reading measures (Word Recognition and Reading Composite) there is no evidence for a significant h_g^2 at any level of disability. For example, the values of h_g^2 for Word Recognition are given in Table 4 and none of these is significant at $P < 0.05$. However spelling especially when IQ is controlled showed more substantial values of h_g^2 (Table 5). When the reading process measures are considered, Phonological Coding shows a consistently high h_g^2 across all levels of severity but is only significant when the most extreme disability group with IQ controlled is analysed (Table 6). Orthographic Coding shows no significant values of h_g^2; the values are negative but not significantly different from zero (Table 7). It should be noted that standard errors for the Orthographic Coding measures are large. To obtain a cleaner measure of orthographic ability, the irregular/exception word reading scores were regressed onto the Phonological Coding scores. The resultant residuals were subjected to a multiple regression analysis to estimate h_g^2. It was found that the measure of Orthographic Coding with Phonological Coding controlled produced values of h_g^2 using 0.5, 1.0 and 1.5 standard deviation definitions of probands that were not significantly different from zero (−0.45, −0.49, −0.91 and respectively). The most consistent results concern the measure of Homophone Recognition, e.g. do "bored" and "board" sound the same. Here the values of h_g^2 are consistently above 0.5 and are significantly greater than zero in all but one case (Table 8).

These results give credence to phonological abilities being the mediator of the genetic influences. The measures of Orthographic Coding do not

Table 4. The heritability of group membership ($B_2 = h_g^2$) for Schonell Single Word Reading Test (Word Recognition) using probands at 0.5, 1.0 and 1.5 standard deviations below mean with and without IQ controlled

Proband	N Probands		Probands				Co-Twins							
			MZ		DZ		MZ		DZ					
Definition	MZ	DZ	Mean	SD	Mean	SD	Mean	SD	Mean	SD	B_1	SE	B_2	SE
Without IQ Controlled														
0.5	40	67	−1.11	0.52	−1.53	0.80	−0.73	0.80	−0.80	1.22	0.31	0.19	0.26	0.38
1.0	23	42	−1.45	0.42	−2.01	0.62	−0.69	0.96	−0.92	1.31	0.59*	0.34	0.03	0.37
1.5	9	32	−1.86	0.37	−2.24	0.51	−0.37	1.07	−1.19	1.27	0.90*	0.43	−0.66	0.46
With IQ Controlled														
0.5	51	62	−1.14	0.66	−1.37	0.72	−0.60	0.76	−0.44	1.15	0.16	0.15	0.41	0.33
1.0	20	38	−1.72	0.71	−1.77	0.63	−0.66	0.82	−0.65	1.19	0.03	0.24	0.03	0.37
2.0	10	23	−2.23	0.69	−2.12	0.57	−0.50	1.00	−0.65	1.28	0.16	0.39	−0.16	0.46

Scores have been standardised in relation to the total sample mean and standard deviation
* $P < 0.05$.

Table 5. The heritability of group membership ($B_2 = h_g^2$) for Schonell Spelling Test using probands at 0.5, 1.0 and 1.5 standard deviations below mean with and without IQ controlled

			Probands				Co-Twins							
Proband	N Probands		MZ		DZ		MZ		DZ					
Definition	MZ	DZ	Mean	SD	Mean	SD	Mean	SD	Mean	SD	B_1	SE	B_2	SE
Without IQ Controlled														
0.5	48	69	−0.96	0.36	−1.42	0.73	−0.67	0.63	−0.72	1.16	0.56**	0.16	0.39	0.32
1.0	19	43	−1.32	0.27	−1.82	0.66	−0.93	0.65	−0.85	1.10	0.72***	0.24	0.47	0.33
1.5	3	25	−1.76	0.28	−2.27	0.48	−0.86	0.34	−1.20	1.21	1.02*	0.50	−0.08	0.65
With IQ Controlled														
0.5	48	61	−1.20	0.49	−1.32	0.62	−0.82	0.78	−0.44	1.05	0.46**	0.17	0.69*	0.32
1.0	30	38	−1.48	0.40	−1.67	0.53	−0.98	0.84	−0.62	1.04	0.34	0.30	0.58*	0.34
1.5	11	19	−1.92	0.29	−2.06	0.48	−1.28	1.05	−0.69	1.22	0.31	0.59	0.66	0.49

Scores have been standardised in relation to the total sample mean and standard deviation
* $P < 0.05$, ** $P < 0.01$, *** $P < 0.001$.

Table 6. The heritability of group membership ($B_2 = h_g^2$) for Non-Words Aloud (Phonological Coding) using probands at 0.5, 1.0 and 1.5 standard deviations above mean with and without IQ controlled

Proband	N Probands		Probands				Co-Twins							
			MZ		DZ		MZ		DZ					
Definition	MZ	DZ	Mean	SD	Mean	SD	Mean	SD	Mean	SD	B_1	SE	B_2	SE
Without IQ Controlled														
0.5	51	58	1.16	0.73	1.49	0.99	0.74	1.08	0.67	1.31	0.39**	0.16	0.37	0.40
1.0	27	36	1.62	0.73	2.03	0.89	1.08	1.12	0.93	1.27	0.24	0.22	0.41	0.39
1.5	7	22	2.63	0.77	2.54	0.78	2.04	1.15	1.14	1.27	−0.65	0.33	0.65	0.46
With IQ Controlled														
0.5	47	47	1.34	0.73	1.59	0.86	0.80	1.04	0.50	1.27	0.21	0.17	0.56	0.37
1.0	30	35	1.70	0.69	1.88	0.81	0.89	1.12	0.65	1.31	0.03	0.24	0.36	0.39
1.5	15	21	2.15	0.73	2.32	0.76	1.25	1.25	0.39	1.23	0.06	0.31	0.82*	0.41

Scores have been standardised in relation to the total sample mean and standard deviation
* $P < 0.05$, ** $P < 0.01$, *** $P < 0.001$.

Table 7. The heritability of group membership ($B_2 = h_g^2$) for Irregular Word Aloud (Orthographic Coding) using probands at 0.5, 1.0 and 1.5 standard deviations above mean with and without IQ controlled

Proband Definition	N Probands MZ	N Probands DZ	Probands MZ Mean	Probands MZ SD	Probands DZ Mean	Probands DZ SD	Co-Twins MZ Mean	Co-Twins MZ SD	Co-Twins DZ Mean	Co-Twins DZ SD	B_1	SE	B_2	SE
Without IQ Controlled														
0.5	22	53	1.10	0.64	1.78	1.14	0.27	0.68	0.84	1.45	0.34	0.32	−0.45	0.42
1.0	6	30	1.91	0.77	2.52	1.01	0.03	0.73	1.18	1.54	0.54*	0.25	−0.91	0.53
1.5	3	23	2.45	0.76	2.90	0.83	0.09	0.93	1.25	1.59	0.97**	0.35	−0.79	0.61
With IQ Controlled														
0.5	28	50	1.11	0.71	1.74	1.15	0.33	0.63	0.63	1.48	0.25*	0.14	−0.12	0.38
1.0	9	35	1.90	0.82	2.17	1.12	0.10	0.61	0.85	1.69	0.38*	0.22	−0.68	0.56
1.5	6	20	2.26	0.77	2.90	0.96	0.08	0.60	1.07	1.94	0.52	0.38	−0.66	0.59

Scores have been standardised in relation to the total sample mean and standard deviation
* $P < 0.05$, ** $P < 0.01$, *** $P < 0.001$.

Table 8. The heritability of group membership ($B_2 = h_g^2$) for Homophone Recognition using probands at 0.5, 1.0 and 1.5 standard deviations above mean with and without IQ controlled

Proband Definition	N Probands MZ	N Probands DZ	Probands MZ Mean	Probands MZ SD	Probands DZ Mean	Probands DZ SD	Co-Twins MZ Mean	Co-Twins MZ SD	Co-Twins DZ Mean	Co-Twins DZ SD	B_1	SE	B_2	SE
Without IQ Controlled														
0.5	40	54	1.24	0.52	1.63	0.90	0.90	0.85	0.51	1.22	0.36*	0.19	0.83***	0.33
1.0	23	35	1.60	0.35	2.13	0.71	1.11	0.82	0.67	1.36	0.33	0.30	0.75*	0.36
1.5	13	26	1.85	0.24	2.41	0.61	1.38	0.61	0.85	1.41	−0.14	0.44	0.78*	0.39
With IQ Controlled														
0.5	41	53	1.28	0.57	1.47	0.85	0.65	0.80	0.25	1.14	0.29*	0.15	0.67**	0.32
1.0	25	33	1.61	0.49	1.94	0.75	0.80	0.88	0.34	1.30	0.33	0.24	0.64*	0.35
1.5	16	22	1.85	0.45	2.29	0.67	0.90	0.98	0.45	1.50	0.31	0.39	0.59	0.43

Scores have been standardised in relation to the total sample mean and standard deviation
* $P < 0.05$, ** $P < 0.01$, *** $P < 0.001$.

show the pattern of sustained h_g^2 across the range, whereas Phonological Coding and the tests concerned with identifying rhyming written words and non-words have consistently high values of h_g^2.

WHICH ASPECTS OF THE READING PROCESS ARE AFFECTED?

The identification of which aspects of the reading process are most strongly influenced by genetic factors is crucially dependent upon the model of reading that is addressed. The reading tasks that have been the subject of genetic analyses in this paper are all single words or letter strings. This restricts their implications to aspects of word naming and leaves aside issues concerned with semantics and comprehension of text.

This was planned using the model of dual route processing (Coltheart, 1978). Indeed the reading tasks that were used were developed by Max Coltheart to test individual differences in the processing within the dual route model. The clear implication of the present findings are that individual differences in the functioning of the phonological route, as measured by non-word reading, are affected by genetic differences between children. Variance in lexical route functioning shows no heritability.

This dual route model has been the subject of a number of critiques. Initially the notion of grapheme-phoneme correspondence rules was criticised. It was argued that larger sub-lexical units could be used to generate a phonological code (Marcel, 1980, Henderson, 1982). These analogy theories retain the lexical route and cannot be differentiated within the present data from the original dual route model. Under either of these theoretical formulations it is the generation of the phonological code by whatever means that carries the genetic effect.

A more radical reformulated model of word naming is that put forward by Shallice and McCarthy (1985). Humphreys and Evett (1985) give this as an example of a more general class of multiple-levels approaches (see also Van Orden, Pennington and Stone, in press). These abandon the simple distinction and independence of lexical and grapheme based processes. Rather letter strings are processed in parallel at several levels between single letters and whole words. It further allows lexical information to influence the processing of all letter units and letters strings, including non-words. Within this framework the present findings suggest that it is those parts of the process that require most word specific knowledge (i.e. exception words) that are less influenced by genetic effects.

The high heritability of phonologically based competencies also marries well with the structure of recent parallel distributed processing models. These have modeled aspects of the acquisition of reading skill (Seidenberg and McClelland, 1987) and features of acquired dyslexia (Patterson, Seidenberg and McClelland, 1989). It is too early to seek to develop strong analogies between features of these computational procedures and biological systems. However it could be suggested that genetic effects may be mediated via an impact on the systems architecture e.g. in terms of the number of "hidden units". These PDP models differ from the dual route formulation by having no direct lexical route. Instead recognition of irregular or exception words comes as a by product of the application of specific learning rules to written inputs. If the twin data had shown strong genetic effects on the reading irregularly spelt words this would not have fitted the PDP model so well.

However as Baron (1985) has argued these detailed concerns with the possible alternative processes in reading single words have lost sight of more salient questions that touch upon the process of reading acquisition. He suggests that more appropriate questions about word recognition might be "Do we need to teach children to decode words they have never seen before? Does such novel-word decoding play a role only in learning or in fluent reading as well?" This leads to research questions such as whether there are separate mechanisms for reading non-words (a surrogate for novel words) and for familiar words. He suggests that the evidence is clear that there are separate pathways that are used simultaneously in word naming and that this happens even in fluent reading (Baron, 1977; Treiman, Freyd and Baron, 1983). Fitting the present findings into Baron's account leads to the conclusion that the genetic-based difficulty with non-word reading will have a marked initial and then an enduring impact on the later reading competence of affected children. This leads to the need to consider in more detail different aspects of such phonological processing.

PHONOLOGICAL DISABILITY AND READING

A number of studies lend support to the notion that phonological disability lies at the root of most children's reading disability. Concurrent and relatively specific deficits in phonological processing have been found in such children (see Wagner and Torgesen, 1987 for a review). It has been suggested (Ehri, 1989) that these phonological abilities are a product rather than a cause of reading disability. She further argues that this effect is mediated by the failure to acquire appropriate spelling knowledge.

However a strong case for the reciprocal interaction in the development of phonological ability, reading and spelling has been made by Goswami and Bryant (1990). They suggest that there are separate contributions to literacy that come from processes based upon phonemic awareness and from the ability to detect rhyme. Their model proposes that success at reading is influenced both directly by an ability to detect rhymes and by an awareness of phonemes. For spelling there was no evidence of a direct effect of rhymes on spelling although differences in rhyming were related to later phonemic awareness.

If Goswami and Bryant are correct it might be expected that these two separate phonological abilities might have some echoes in later reading ability. It is of interest therefore to return to the measures of Phonological Coding and Homophone Recognition to establish whether these represent indices of some common underlying ability to process the phonological characteristics of words or whether distinct abilities are involved. These two measures were correlated at $r = 0.608$ ($P < 0.001$).

For the total sample the Phonological Coding score obtained from non-word reading was regressed onto the child's Homophone Recognition score. The standardised residuals were derived and were found to be uncorrelated with IQ ($r = 0.013$, ns). The reverse regression was also undertaken predicting Homophone Recognition from Phonological Coding. This residual was found to be correlated with IQ ($r = -0.431$, $P < 0.01$). Accordingly IQ was added to the regression equation to generate residuals independent of both IQ and Phonological Coding. These residual scores are still based upon errors so that Phonological Coding (based upon letter to sound correspondences in non-word reading) and Homophone Recognition (assumed to be tapping some aspects of rhyme recognition since homophone judgment could be considered to the most extreme form of rhyme detection) would be expected to negatively correlated with Word Recognition ($r = -0.186$, $P < 0.05$ and $r = -0.371$, $P < 0.01$ respectively).

As would be expected from the way the scores were derived there is a negative correlation between them ($r = -0.638$, $P < 0.001$). When probands are identified at -1.00 standard deviation only one child was in both groups. These probands are 59 cases where non-word reading is poor in relation to what would be expected from their Homophone recognition and 57 cases whose Homophone Recognition is poorer than would be expected given their non-word reading. In both cases proband membership is independent of IQ.

If these two aspects of phonological ability are reflecting a common underlying characteristic these residuals are likely to reflect non-systematic effects and to show little evidence of heritability. On the other hand if there were distinct abilities in addition to any common competencies then either one or possibly both will show a significant heritability. In the same way as before the estimation of h_g^2 can be obtained at varying degrees of severity. The results for Non-word reading with Homophone Recognition controlled are given in Table 9. Significant values of h_g^2 are obtained in each case. For Homophone Recognition with Non-word and IQ controlled, the results were less clear (Table 10). A significant h_g^2 is obtained only with the most extreme cases.

A further check on whether these are independent aspects of *phono-*

Table 9. The heritability of group membership ($B_2 = h_g^2$) for Non-word Reading using probands at 0.5, 1.0 and 1.5 standard deviations above mean with homophone recognition controlled

			Probands				Co-Twins							
Proband	N Probands		MZ		DZ		MZ		DZ					
Definition	MZ	DZ	Mean	SD	Mean	SD	Mean	SD	Mean	SD	B_1	SE	B_2	SE
0.5	52	40	1.34	0.79	1.51	0.78	0.56	1.12	0.17	1.13	0.24	0.17	0.61$	0.33
1.0	32	27	1.75	0.74	1.89	0.66	0.84	1.21	0.05	1.00	0.14	0.24	0.91**	0.38
1.5	18	17	2.17	0.74	2.27	0.54	0.81	1.40	−0.03	0.99	0.35	0.34	0.74*	0.39

Scores have been standardised in relation to the total sample mean and standard deviation
$ $P < 0.06$, * $P < 0.05$, ** $P < 0.01$, *** $P < 0.001$.

Table 10. The heritability of group membership ($B_2 = h_g^2$) for Homophone Recognition using probands at 0.5, 1.0 and 1.5 standard deviations above mean with non-word reading and IQ controlled

			Probands				Co-Twins							
Proband	N Probands		MZ		DZ		MZ		DZ					
Definition	MZ	DZ	Mean	SD	Mean	SD	Mean	SD	Mean	SD	B_1	SE	B_2	SE
0.5	37	60	1.11	0.59	1.46	0.87	0.51	0.98	0.33	1.17	−0.09	0.17	0.47	0.35
1.0	15	36	1.62	0.63	1.92	0.85	0.41	1.22	0.20	1.14	0.07	0.23	0.29	0.39
1.5	7	22	2.07	0.66	2.38	0.77	1.07	1.09	0.09	1.20	0.95*	0.47	0.74*	0.39

Scores have been standardised in relation to the total sample mean and standard deviation
* $P < 0.05$, ** $P < 0.01$, *** $P < 0.001$.

logical ability was made. It could be argued that since the Homophone Recognition task is based upon non-word, regular and irregular word reading, the measure could be sensitive to variation in orthographic ability. The Homophone Recognition scores were therefore regressed onto Orthographic Coding (irregular word reading) as well as non-word reading and IQ. The results indicated that a rather higher level of h_g^2 was obtained when orthographic ability was controlled i.e. 0.86 ($P < 0.01$), 0.75 ($P < 0.05$), and 0.71 (ns) for 0.5, 1.0 and 1.5 standard deviation definitions of proband respectively.

Overall these results indicate that there are possibly two distinct aspects of phonological ability being tapped by these measures. The one that is concerned with letter-sound correspondences in non-word reading shows consistent evidence for genetic influences. A separate group of individuals can be identified who show specific Homophone Recognition deficits; the data is consistent with genetic effects contributing to these deficits. These effects are even stronger when Orthographic Coding ability is controlled.

These reading tasks are different from the phoneme recognition and rhyme and alliteration tasks used by Goswami and Bryant (1990). But if they do reflect analogies to these components of phonological skill that are present in the reading abilities of older children both components show influences of genetic factors. However it must be emphasized again that at age thirteen these genetic effects are less salient for overall reading ability and are shown most strongly in spelling ability.

CONCLUSIONS

It is clear that the Colorado and London twin reading studies, despite their very different methodologies, are in agreement in identifying phonological ability as the most likely mediator of genetic influences on reading ability. These genetic effects are not simply a by-product of more general genetic influences on intelligence. The task is now to undertake genuinely developmental twin studies to establish the links between genetic influences on early language processing and later literacy.

The results presented in the present paper compliment the phonological-core variable difference model of Stanovich (1988). The analyses clearly identify a dimensional approach to reading and spelling difficulties as being appropriate; for example by the maintenance of similar group heritability at all levels of disability. Secondly it identifies a major contribution or rather contributions to the phonological core as stemming from genetic variance between children.

At first sight, the results may appear to fit less well with studies suggesting that single major gene effects may play a part in causing reading disabilities. As was emphasized earlier, a sustained level of heritability of deviant group membership across a range of severity of disability does not necessarily indicate that the same genetic mechanisms are acting at all levels of disability. It is possible that single major genes are influencing disability at the more extreme end of the range and that other possibly polygenic mechanisms account for individual differences within the more normal range. This is an unconvincing explanation since it assumes that just by chance these two mechanism happen to produce similar values of h_g^2 at different parts of the range. A more parsimonious explanation is that for the vast majority of children variation in reading ability is influenced by a polygenic system or systems that have an impact via possibly two aspects phonological ability. For a much smaller proportion of the population of disabled readers major gene effects are acting. These latter cases are simply too rare to effect the results of the London twin study. Their scarcity is indicated by the problem of identifying suitable pedigrees for linkage analyses (Smith et al., in press).

The findings from the present study highlight the need for a longitudinal study of reading development in a large representative samples of twins. The following predictions can be made about the outcome of such a study. At younger ages the heritability of spelling will be unchanged and the heritability of reading will be higher and would be more consistent across levels of reading disability in the younger age groups. Such a study would also permit the exploration of a more developmentally oriented framework for reading disability. If genetic factors are playing a significant role in the acquisition of various aspects of phonological ability in children (Goswami and Bryant, 1990), this should have a discernible and relatively specific impact on developmental processes such as those proposed by Frith (1985). Longitudinal twin data could provide a crucial test of the validity of such a theoretical formulation.

ACKNOWLEDGEMENTS

This study was supported by a grant from the Medical Research Council, U.K. to Professor Philip Graham (Institute for Child Health, London) and the author. I would like thank Professor John DeFries for his clarification of the sampling implications of double and single entry regression analysis. Dick Olson kindly provided access to some of the as yet unpublished findings from the Colorado Reading Project. I am also grateful for his incisive comments on an earlier draft of the paper. I would like to thank Keith Stanovich for suggesting additional analyses to clarify the results for phonological and orthographic coding. Jackie Gillis provided valuable guidance on the correction of the standard errors.

Genetic Etiology of Spelling Deficits in the Colorado and London Twin Studies of Reading Disability

J. C. DEFRIES,[1] JIM STEVENSON,[2] JACQUELYN J. GILLIS [1] and SALLY J. WADSWORTH[1]

[1] *Institute for Behavioral Genetics, University of Colorado, Boulder, CO 80309, U.S.A.*
[2] *Department of Psychology, University of Surrey, Guildford, Surrey GU2 5XH, U.K.*

ABSTRACT: The basic multiple regression model for the analysis of selected twin data (DeFries and Fulker 1985, 1988) was fitted to spelling data from 100 pairs of MZ twins and 71 pairs of same-sex DZ twins tested in the Colorado Reading Project (DeFries, Olson, Pennington and Smith 1991), and to data from 12 pairs of MZ twins and 15 pairs of same-sex DZ twins tested in the London twin study of reading disability (Stevenson, Graham, Fredman and McLoughlin 1984, 1987). Estimates of h_g^2 obtained from analyses of these data suggest that about 60% of the deficit of probands is due to heritable influences in both samples. When a regression model was fitted separately to data from males and females in the combined Colorado and London samples, resulting estimates of h_g^2 were 0.66 ± 0.18 and 0.56 ± 0.19, respectively, a nonsignificant difference. Collaborative analyses of data from additional twin studies of reading disability would facilitate more rigorous tests of hypotheses of differential genetic etiology as a function of group membership.

KEYWORDS: Spelling, reading disability, genetics, etiology, twins.

Previous twin studies of reading disability (Zerbin-Rüdin 1967, Bakwin 1973, and Stevenson, Graham, Fredman and McLoughlin 1984 and 1987) employed a comparison of concordance rates in identical (monozygotic, MZ) and fraternal (dizygotic, DZ) twin pairs as a test for genetic etiology. A pair is concordant if both members of the pair manifest a condition, but discordant if only one member is affected. Thus, a genetic etiology is indicated if the MZ concordance rate for a condition exceeds that for DZ twin pairs.

Although the concept for concordance is conceptually very simple, its estimation is dependent upon the method of sample ascertainment. For example, if a sample of twins is ascertained by "single selection" in which only one member of a pair could be selected as a proband, then "pairwise" concordance is appropriate. However, if "truncate selection" is employed in which both affected members of a twin pair could be ascertained as probands, then "probandwise" concordance should be computed. To estimate probandwise concordance, members of concordant pairs are counted twice, once as a proband and once as a cotwin (see DeFries and Gillis, 1991). Because subjects in previous twin studies of reading dis-

Reading and Writing: An Interdisciplinary Journal 3: 271–283, 1991.
© 1991 *Kluwer Academic Publishers.*

ability were likely ascertained employing truncate selection, probandwise concordance rates will be reported in this brief review.

Concordance Rates in Twin Studies of Reading Disability

Zerbin-Rüdin (1967) reviewed data from six case studies of twins with "congenital word-blindness" (5 MZ pairs and 1 DZ pair), a Danish twin study (Norrie 1954, Hermann and Norrie 1958) that included 9 MZ and 30 DZ pairs, and data from 3 MZ and 3 DZ twin pairs included in Hallgren's (1950) classic family study of dyslexia. In this combined sample of 17 pairs of identical twins and 34 pairs of fraternal twins, the probandwise concordance rates are 100% and 52%, respectively. Bakwin (1973) ascertained pairs of same-sex twins through mothers-of-twins clubs and obtained reading history information from parents via interviews, telephone calls, and mail questionnaires. In 31 pairs of identical twins and 31 pairs of fraternal twins in which at least one member of each pair met his criterion for reading disability, the probandwise concordance rates are 91% and 45%. Although these two early publications are based upon data from very different samples, it is interesting to note that their estimated probandwise concordance rates are highly similar.

More recently, Stevenson et al. (1984, 1987) reported results from the first twin study of reading disability in which twin pairs were ascertained from the general population and independently tested using standardized measures of intelligence and of reading and spelling performance. A sample of 285 pairs of 13-year-old twins was obtained by screening hospital records in five London boroughs or through primary schools in the London area. Twins were diagnosed for reading or spelling "backwardness" or "retardation," where backwardness was identified by the presence of reading or spelling performance below that expected based on chronological age, and retardation was defined by marked underachievement in reading or spelling relative to that predicted from IQ and chronological age. Probandwise concordance rates employing these various diagnostic criteria ranged from 33% to 59% for MZ twins and from 29% to 54% for fraternal twins. Stevenson et al. (1987) speculated that the lower concordance rates for reading disability obtained in the London study may have been due to differences in age of subjects, method of sample ascertainment, definition of disability, or zygosity determination.

A more extensive twin study of reading disability was initiated in 1982 as part of the ongoing Colorado Reading Project (Decker and Vandenberg 1985, DeFries 1985). A psychometric test battery that includes the WISC-R (1974) or the Wechsler Adult Intelligence Scale-Revised (WAIS-R; Wechsler 1981) and the Peabody Individual Achievement Test (PIAT; Dunn and Markwardt 1970) is currently being administered to MZ and

DZ twin pairs in which at least one member of each pair is reading disabled and to a comparison group of twins with no history of reading problems. In a recent report (DeFries and Gillis 1991) data from the PIAT Reading Recognition, Reading Comprehension, and Spelling subtests were used to compute a discriminant function score for each member of the pair. Twin pairs were included in the proband sample if at least one member of the pair with a positive school history for reading problems was classified as affected by the discriminant score and met additional criteria for proband diagnosis. In a sample of 96 pairs of MZ twins, 72 pairs of same-sex DZ twins, and 24 pairs of opposite-sex DZ twins in which at least one member of each pair met the criteria for reading disability, the probandwise MZ and DZ concordance rates were 71% and 49%, respectively.

Multiple Regression Analysis of Twin Data

Although a comparison of concordance rates is appropriate for categorical variables (e.g., presence or absence of a disease state), reading disability is diagnosed on the basis of a continuous measure such as reading or spelling performance with arbitrary cut-off points (Stevenson et al. 1987). For such variables, a comparison of MZ and DZ cotwin means is more appropriate than a comparison of concordance rates as a test for genetic etiology (DeFries and Fulker 1985). When probands have been ascertained because of highly deviant scores on a continuous measure, the scores of both the MZ and DZ cotwins should regress toward the mean of the unselected population. However, to the extent that the condition has a genetic etiology, scores of DZ cotwins should regress more toward the mean of the unselected population. Thus, if the means for the MZ and DZ probands were equal, a *t*-test of the difference between the means of the MZ and DZ cotwins would suffice as a test for genetic etiology. However, fitting a multiple regression model to selected twin data, in which the cotwin's score is predicted from the proband's score and the coefficient of relationship, provides a more general and statistically more powerful test (DeFries and Fulker 1985, 1988). Moreover, a simple transformation of twin data prior to multiple regression analysis facilitates direct estimates of h_g^2, an index of the extent to which the deficit of probands is due to heritable influences. For example, DeFries and Gillis (1991) obtained an estimate of $h_g^2 = 0.50 \pm 0.11$ for a composite measure of reading performance when the multiple regression model was fitted to data from probands and cotwins tested in the Colorado Reading Project. This result suggests that about one-half of the reading performance deficit of probands, on average, is due to heritable factors.

The multiple regression analysis of selected twin data is a highly flexible methodology. For example, the basic model can be easily extended to include other main effects such as age, IQ, or socioeconomic status. Interactions between main effects can also be added to the regression model (Cohen and Cohen 1975) to assess differential genetic etiology as a function of group membership (e.g., sample or gender).

In order to increase the number of reading-disabled MZ and DZ twin pairs available for multiple regression analysis, we have recently initiated a collaborative analysis of data collected in the Colorado and London twin studies of reading disability. Although multiple regression analysis was applied previously to a composite measure of reading performance in the Colorado study (e.g., DeFries, Fulker and LaBuda 1987, DeFries and Gillis 1991), differences between the Colorado and London test batteries made it difficult to create a comparable composite reading measure for the two studies. Stevenson et al. (1984) have previously suggested that genetic influences on literacy problems are more appropriately studied through their impact on spelling than on measures of word recognition or reading comprehension. There are several reasons for postulating that spelling may be less susceptible than reading to environmental influences. First, there is evidence that spelling performance of reading-disabled children improves less over time than does reading (Rutter and Yule 1975, Critchley and Critchley 1978). Second, spelling is a more constrained task than reading. Because there are fewer contextual clues to spelling vis-a-vis word naming, there is a greater scope for remediating reading difficulties. Third, genetic etiology may differ more as a function of age for reading than for spelling deficits (Wadsworth, Gillis, DeFries and Fulker 1989). Thus, in this first report, we focus upon spelling deficits and present estimates of h_g^2 for the current Colorado sample, the London sample, and a pooled estimate obtained from our combined data sets.

Recent studies have indicated that reading-disabled females obtained somewhat higher average spelling scores than males (Vogel 1990, DeFries, Wadsworth and Gillis 1990), and there is some limited evidence for a differential genetic etiology of reading deficits in males and females (DeFries, Gillis and Wadsworth, in press). Allred (1990) has recently discussed gender differences in spelling achievement and suggested that additional information concerning the etiology of these differences is needed. We, therefore, also tested the hypothesis of differential genetic etiology of spelling deficits as a function of gender in the combined sample.

METHOD

Subjects. Twin pairs are identified in the Colorado Reading Project by administrators of school districts within a 150-mile radius of Boulder, Colorado, and permission is then sought from parents to review the school records of both members of each pair for evidence of reading problems. Such evidence includes low reading achievement test scores, referral to resource rooms or reading therapists because of poor reading performance, reports by classroom teachers or school psychologists, and parental interviews (Gillis and DeFries 1989). Pairs of twins in which at least one member has a positive history of a reading problem are then invited to be tested at the University of Colorado where they are administered an extensive test battery that includes the WISC-R (Wechsler 1974) or the WAIS-R (Wechsler 1981) and the Peabody Individual Achievement Test (PIAT; Dunn and Markwardt 1970).

In order to assess the genetic etiology of spelling deficits in the Colorado twin sample, the mean and standard deviation of age-adjusted PIAT Spelling scores of 432 individuals from twin pairs in which neither member of the pair had a positive history of reading problems were first calculated. Pairs of twins were then selected for multiple regression analysis if either member of the pair had a positive history of reading problems, and, in addition, had a spelling score at least one standard deviation below the mean of the controls. Other diagnostic criteria include an IQ score of at least 90 on either the Verbal or Performance Scale of the WISC or WAIS; no diagnosed neurological, emotional, or behavioral problems; and no uncorrected visual or auditory acuity deficits.

Selected items from the Nichols and Bilbro (1966) questionnaire were administered to determine zygosity of same-sex twin pairs. In ambiguous cases, zygosity of the pair was confirmed by analysis of blood samples. The sample of twins ascertained in this manner includes 100 pairs of MZ twins (47 male and 53 female pairs) and 71 pairs of same-sex DZ twins (39 male and 32 female pairs). Subjects ranged in age from 8 to 20 years at the time of testing and all had been reared in English-speaking, middle-class homes.

Subjects in the London twin study were administered a test battery that included the Wechsler Intelligence Scale for Children-Revised (WISC-R; Wechsler 1974), the Neale Analysis of Reading Ability (Neale 1967), and the Schonell Graded Word Reading and Spelling Tests (Schonell and Schonell 1960). The mean and standard deviation of the Schonell Spelling scores of 541 13-year-old children in the London twin sample were computed. Twin pairs in which at least one member of the pair had a spelling score one standard deviation or more below the sample mean and a Verbal or Performance IQ of at least 90 were then selected for multiple regression analysis. Zygosity was assessed using physical similarity criteria and, when necessary, dermatoglyphics and blood-group testing. This sample includes 12 pairs of MZ twins (8 male and 4 female pairs) and 15 pairs of same-sex DZ twins (11 male and 4 female pairs).

Analysis. In order to assess the heritable nature of spelling deficits in the Colorado and London twin studies, the following multiple regression model was fitted separately to the spelling scores of the twins in the two selected samples:

$$C = B_1P + B_2R + A, \quad (1)$$

where C is the expected cotwin's score, P is the proband's score, R is the coefficient of relationship (R = 1.0 for MZ twins and 0.5 for DZ twins), and A is the regression constant. B_1 is the partial regression of cotwin's score on proband's score, i.e., the weighted average of the separate MZ and DZ cotwin-proband regression coefficients. Thus, B_1 estimates the average regression in this sample for twin pairs without regard to zygosity. B_2, the partial regression of cotwin's score on the coefficient of relationship, equals twice the difference between the means of the MZ and DZ cotwins after covariance adjustment for any difference in the average scores of the MZ and DZ probands. To the extent that the deficit of probands is due to heritable influences, MZ and DZ cotwins will regress differentially to the mean of the unselected population. Therefore, B_2 provides a test of significance for genetic etiology. If each subject's score is expressed as a deviation from the control means prior to regression analysis, B_2 yields a direct estimate of h^2_g. Because truncate selection was employed to ascertain these samples of affected twins, pairs concordant for spelling deficits were double entered for all analyses in a manner analogous to that used for computation of probandwise concordance rates, and standard errors of the resulting regression coefficients were adjusted accordingly (see DeFries, Gillis and Wadsworth, in press).

A pooled estimate of h^2_g was then obtained by fitting the following extended regression model to data from the two samples simultaneously:

$$C = B_1P + B_2R + B_3S + A, \quad (2)$$

where S is a dummy variable representing sample (+0.5 for each subject in the Colorado sample and −0.5 for the London sample).

In order to test for a differential genetic etiology of spelling deficits in the two samples, the following model was fitted to the combined data sets:

$$C = B_1P + B_2R + B_3S + B_4PS + B_5RS + A, \quad (3)$$

where PS is the product of proband's score and sample, and where RS is the product of relationship and sample. B_4 tests for differential twin resemblance in the two samples, and B_5 tests the significance of the difference between the estimates of h^2_g obtained from the separate analyses of the two data sets.

In order to assess the possibility of a gender difference in h^2_g for spelling deficits, equation 2 was fitted separately to data from males and females in the combined samples. Finally, the significance of this gender difference was tested by fitting the following model to data from both males and females in the combined data set:

$$C = B_1P + B_2R + B_3S + B_4G + B_5PS + B_6PG + B_7RS + B_8RG + B_9SG + A, \quad (4)$$

where G symbolizes gender (coded +0.5 and −0.5 for males and females, respectively). B_4 estimates the differences between the means of male and female probands and B_5, B_6, B_7, B_8 and B_9 provide tests of significance for the indicated interactions. Although additional interaction terms could be included in equations 3 and 4, we focus upon tests of differential genetic etiology as a function of sample (B_5, equation 3) and gender (B_8, equation 4) in this analysis.

RESULTS

The average spelling scores of the MZ and DZ probands and cotwins in the Colorado sample, expressed in standard deviation units from the mean of 432 control subjects, are presented in Table 1. Average spelling scores of selected twins from the London sample, expressed as standard deviations from the mean of 541 individuals that comprised the unselected sample, are also tabulated. From this table it may be seen that the average spelling scores of MZ and DZ probands in the Colorado sample are similar and about two standard deviations below the mean of the matched comparison sample of unaffected twins. In contrast, the average scores of probands in the London sample are somewhat less deviant, and scores of the MZ probands are higher (i.e., less negative) than those of DZ probands. The difference between the average scores of probands in the

Table 1. Mean spelling scores of selected twin pairs tested in the Colorado and London twin studies of reading disability.

Sample		Proband	Cotwin	N_{Pairs}
Colorado[a]	Identical	−2.01	−1.80	100
	Fraternal	−1.92	−1.13	71
London[b]	Identical	−1.29	−0.97	12
	Fraternal	−1.72	−0.77	15

[a] Expressed as standard deviation units from the mean of 432 control individuals in the Colorado Twin Sample.

[b] Expressed as standard deviation units from the mean of 541 individuals in the unselected London Twin Sample.

two samples is presumably due to the difference in diagnostic criteria employed in the two studies. In the Colorado study, a positive school history of reading problems was an additional ascertainment criterion. The difference in average scores of MZ and DZ twins in the London sample has been previously noted by Stevenson et al. (1987). Nevertheless, it may be seen that scores of the DZ cotwins in both samples have regressed more than those of MZ cotwins toward their respective population means. In the Colorado sample, the scores of the DZ cotwins have regressed 0.79 standard deviation units on the average toward the control mean, whereas those of MZ cotwins have regressed only 0.21 standard deviation units. In the London sample, these cotwin-proband differences for DZ and MZ twins are 0.95 and 0.32 standard deviation units, respectively. This differential regression of MZ and DZ cotwin means toward the unselected population mean clearly suggests a substantial genetic etiology for spelling deficits in these two independent studies.

Results of fitting the basic model (equation 1) to the spelling performance data of the Colorado and London twin samples are summarized in Table 2. The estimate of $B_1 = 0.47 \pm 0.10$ obtained from the Colorado sample is a weighted average of the MZ and DZ cotwin-proband regression coefficients for spelling performance, which are 0.61 ± 0.12 and 0.23 ± 0.17, respectively. Corresponding regression coefficients for the selected MZ and DZ twin pairs in the London sample are -0.43 ± 0.70 and -0.03 ± 0.43, respectively, resulting in a B_1 estimate of -0.14. This unexpected negative estimate is almost certainly due in part to the very small number of twin pairs (12 MZ and 15 DZ) with spelling deficits in the London sample. In contrast, the estimates for $B_2 = h_g^2$ obtained from the Colorado and London data sets are remarkably similar, viz., 0.62 ± 0.14 and 0.61 ± 0.39, respectively. These results suggest that over half the spelling performance deficit of probands in the two samples is due to heritable influences.

Table 2. Fit of basic regression model to transformed spelling scores of selected twin pairs tested in the Colorado and London twin studies of reading disability

Sample	Coefficient	Estimate ± S.E.	t	p[a]
Colorado	B_1	0.47 ± 0.10	4.70	<0.001
	$B_2 = h_g^2$	0.62 ± 0.14	4.43	<0.001
London	B_1	-0.14 ± 0.36	−0.39	<0.35
	$B_2 = h_g^2$	0.61 ± 0.39	1.57	<0.06
Combined	B_1	0.42 ± 0.10	4.29	<0.001
	$B_2 = h_g^2$	0.62 ± 0.13	4.68	<0.001

[a] One-tailed.

Pooled estimates of B_1 and B_2 obtained when equation 2 was fitted simultaneously to the two data sets are also presented in Table 2. As expected, given the difference in sample size between the two data sets, the parameter estimates obtained from the combined data are highly similar to those from the Colorado study.

Although there is obviously no evidence for a differential genetic etiology of spelling deficits in the Colorado and London data sets (0.62 and 0.61, respectively), equation 3 was nonetheless fitted to data from the combined samples to test this hypothesis explicitly. As expected, the regression coefficient that provides a test of the magnitude of this interaction is nonsignificant ($B_5 = 0.003 \pm 0.384$, $t = 0.01$, $p > 0.99$, two-tailed). Because sample was coded +0.5 and −0.5 for the Colorado and London data sets, this coefficient exactly equals the difference between the two h_g^2 estimates, i.e., $0.6165 - 0.6131 = 0.0034$. In contrast to the test for the difference between the two estimates of h_g^2, the regression coefficient that assesses differential twin resemblance in the two samples approaches statistical significance ($B_4 = 0.61 \pm 0.35$, $t = 1.77$, $p < 0.08$, two-tailed).

Estimates of h_g^2 obtained by fitting equation 2 separately to transformed spelling data from male and female twin pairs included in the combined data set are presented in Table 3. The resulting estimate of h_g^2 for males (0.66 ± 0.18, $p < 0.001$, one-tailed) is larger than that for females (0.56 ± 0.19, $p < 0.003$), suggesting that genetic factors may be somewhat more important as a cause of spelling deficits in males than in females. However, the coefficient that tests for differential genetic etiology in males and females ($B_8 = 0.10 \pm 0.27$, $p > 0.50$, two-tailed) is not significant.

DISCUSSION

DeFries and Fulker (1985, 1988) have noted that a multiple regression analysis of continuous data from selected twin pairs provides a more

Table 3. Estimates of group heritability of spelling deficits for males and females in the combined Colorado and London data sets

	Number of twin pairs			
Gender	MZ	DZ	$B_2 = h_g^2$	p[a]
Males	55	50	0.66 ± 0.18	<0.001
Females	57	36	0.56 ± 0.19	<0.003

[a] One-tailed.

general and flexible test of genetic etiology than does the comparison of concordance rates employed in previous twin studies (Zerbin-Rüdin 1967, Bakwin 1973, Stevenson et al. 1984, 1987). When probands are identified because of deviant scores on a continuous variable such as reading or spelling performance, genetic factors are implicated if the MZ and DZ cotwin scores regress differentially toward the mean of the unselected population. The partial regression of cotwin's score on the coefficient of relationship (equation 1) estimates twice the difference between the MZ and DZ cotwin means after covariance adjustment for any difference between the MZ and DZ proband means. When each score is transformed by expressing it as a deviation from the mean of the unselected population and dividing by the difference between the proband and control means, this regression coefficient directly estimates h_g^2, an index of the extent to which the deficit of probands is due to heritable influences.

In order to increase the number of twin pairs available for multiple regression analysis, we have combined data collected in the Colorado Reading Project and the London Twin Study. Due to differences between the measures obtained in the Colorado and London studies, the current analyses focus specifically on spelling performance. When equation 1 was fitted to transformed spelling scores from selected MZ and DZ twin pairs in the Colorado and London samples, resulting estimates of h_g^2 were 0.62 ± 0.14 and 0.61 ± 0.39, respectively, suggesting that over half of the deficit in the spelling performance of probands is due to heritable influences in both samples. The similarity between these h_g^2 estimates is remarkable, given the differences between the two studies. Subjects in the Colorado study are administered a test of spelling recognition, whereas subjects in the London study were required to generate correct spellings of individual words. Moreover, different ascertainment criteria were employed to select probands in the two studies. That similar h_g^2 estimates were obtained in these two independent twin studies strengthens the evidence for a substantial genetic etiology of spelling deficits. These estimates of h_g^2 for spelling are somewhat higher than that for a composite measure of reading performance (0.50) estimated from data of the Colorado study (DeFries and Gillis 1991), thus supporting the suggestion of Stevenson et al. (1984) that spelling may be less susceptible than reading to environmental influences.

Multiple regression analysis was also used to test the hypothesis that the cause or causes of spelling disability may differ in males and females. When equation 2 was fitted separately to spelling data from male and female twin pairs in the combined data set, resulting estimates of h_g^2 were 0.66 ± 0.18 and 0.56 ± 0.19, respectively, a nonsignificant difference. Nonetheless, it is interesting to note that the gender difference in estimates of h_g^2 for spelling is opposite that found for a composite measure of reading performance in the Colorado Reading Project (DeFries, Gillis and

Wadsworth, in press). Although the difference in estimates of h_g^2 for reading performance of males and females (0.42 and 0.48, respectively) was also nonsignificant, this differential pattern of results is consistent with the hypothesis of a developmental dissociation between reading and spelling deficits in learning-disabled children (Stevenson et al. 1987, Wadsworth et al. 1989).

The test of genetic etiology provided by the multiple regression analysis of selected twin data is also statistically powerful (DeFries and Fulker 1988). For example, when equation 1 was recently fitted to transformed discriminant function data from the Colorado sample of reading-disabled probands and cotwins (DeFries, Olson, Pennington and Smith 1991), the squared multiple correlation was 0.26 and the correlation between proband and cotwin scores was 0.43. Thus, the power (Cohen 1977) to detect a significant B_2 at the 0.05 level (one-tailed test) in a sample of 100 pairs of MZ and 100 pairs of DZ twins is 0.99. This power of the multiple regression analysis of selected twin data is clearly demonstrated in the present analysis of data from the London twin sample (only 12 pairs of MZ twins and 15 pairs of DZ twins) in which the estimate of h_g^2 is marginally significant ($p < 0.06$, one-tailed).

Because the multiple regression test for genetic etiology is statistically powerful, the test for differential genetic etiology is also relatively powerful. For example, if h_g^2 in males and females differed by 0.5, the power to detect a significant interaction between zygosity and gender at the 0.05 level (two-tailed test) in a sample of 100 pairs of MZ and 100 pairs of DZ twins would be about 0.75 (DeFries and Fulker 1988). However, if the difference in h_g^2 were 0.3, the power would be only about 0.30. By increasing the sample size to 150 pairs of MZ twins and 150 pairs of DZ twins, the power would be increased to about 0.90 and 0.50 in these two cases. Thus, a larger sample of twins will be required to test more rigorously the hypothesis that the etiology of spelling deficits differs as a function of group membership.

Twin studies of reading disability are relatively easy to initiate, and small studies could be readily accomplished even by research groups with limited resources. Results of such twin studies could be individually informative; moreover, collaborative analyses of combined data sets from such studies could facilitate statistically powerful tests of hypotheses that are relevant to several current issues in the field of reading disability (DeFries and Gillis 1991).

ACKNOWLEDGEMENTS

This work was supported in part by program project and center grants from NICHD (HD-11681 and HD-27802) to J. C. DeFries and a project grant from the U.K. Medical Research Council to P. Graham (Institute of Child Health, London) and J. Stevenson. The report was prepared while J. C. DeFries was supported by a University of Colorado Faculty Fellowship and J. Gillis was supported by NIMH training grant MH-16880. The invaluable contributions of staff members of the Colorado and London studies, and of the families who participated in these studies, are gratefully acknowledged. We also thank Rebecca G. Miles for expert editorial assistance.

REFERENCES

Allred, R. A. 1990. Gender differences in spelling achievement in grades 1 through 6. *Journal of Education Research, 83,* 187—193.

Bakwin, H. 1973. Reading disability in twins. *Developmental Medicine and Child Neurology, 15,* 184—187.

Cohen, J. 1977. *Statistical power analysis for the behavioral sciences.* New York: Academic Press.

Cohen, J. and Cohen, P. 1975. *Applied multiple regression/correlation analysis for the behavioral sciences.* New York: Halstead Press.

Critchley, M. and Critchley, E. A. 1978. *Dyslexia defined.* London: Heinemann.

Decker, S. N. and Vandenberg, S. G. 1985. Colorado twin study of reading disability. *In* D. B. Gray and J. F. Kavanagh (eds), *Biobehavioral measures of dyslexia* (pp. 123—135). Parkton, MD: York Press.

DeFries, J. C. 1985. Colorado reading project. *In* D. B. Gray and J. F. Kavanagh (eds), *Biobehavioral measures of dyslexia* (pp. 107—122). Parkton, MD: York Press.

DeFries, J. C. and Fulker, D. W. 1985. Multiple regression analysis of twin data. *Behavior Genetics, 15,* 467—473.

DeFries, J. C. and Fulker, D. W. 1988. Multiple regression analysis of twin data: Etiology of deviant scores versus individual differences. *Acta Geneticae Medicae et Gemellologiae, 37,* 205—216.

DeFries, J. C., Fulker, D. W. and LaBuda, M. C. 1987. Evidence for a genetic aetiology in reading disability of twins. *Nature, 329,* 537—539.

DeFries, J. C. and Gillis, J. J. 1991. Etiology of reading deficits in learning disabilities: Quantitative genetic analysis. *In* J. E. Obrzut and G. W. Hynd (eds), *Neuropsychological foundations of learning disabilities: A Handbook of issues, methods and practice.* Orlando, FL: Academic Press.

DeFries, J. C., Gillis, J. J. and Wadsworth, S. J. (in press). Genes and genders: A twin study of reading disability. *In* A. M. Galaburda (ed), *The extraordinary brain: Neurobiologic issues in developmental dyslexia.* Cambridge, MA: Harvard University Press.

DeFries, J. C., Olson, R. K., Pennington, B. F. and Smith, S. D. 1991. Colorado Reading Project: An update. In D. B. Gray and D. Duane (eds), *The reading brain: The biological basis of dyslexia.* Parkton, MD: York Press.

DeFries, J. C., Wadsworth, S. J. and Gillis, J. J. 1990. Gender differences in cognitive abilities of reading-disabled twins. *Annals of Dyslexia, 40,* 216—228.

Dunn, L. M. and Markwardt, F. C. 1970. *Examiner's manual: Peabody Individual Achievement Test.* Circle Pines, MN: American Guidance Service.

Gillis, J. J. and DeFries, J. C. 1989. Validity of school history as a diagnostic criterion for reading disability. *Reading and Writing: An Interdisciplinary Journal, 1,* 93—101.

Hallgren, B. 1950. Specific dyslexia: A clinical and genetic study. *Acta Psychiatrica and Neurologica Scandinavica, Supplement, 65,* 1—287.

Hermann, K. and Norrie, E. 1958. Is congenital word-blindness an hereditary type of Gerstmann's syndrome? *Psychiatric Neurology, 136*, 59—73.

Neale, M. D. 1967. *Neale analysis of reading ability.* London: Macmillan.

Nichols, R. C. and Bilbro, W. C. 1966. The diagnosis of twin zygosity. *Acta Genetica et Statistica Medica, 16*, 265—275.

Norrie, E. 1954. Ordblindhedens (dyslexiens) arvegang. *Laesepaedagogen, 2*, 61.

Rutter, M. and Yule, W. 1975. The concept of specific reading retardation. *Journal of Child Psychology and Psychiatry, 16*, 181—197.

Schonell, F. J. and Schonell, P. E. 1960. *Diagnostic and attainment testing.* Edinburgh: Oliver & Boyd.

Stevenson, J., Graham, P., Fredman, G. and McLoughlin, V. 1984. The genetics of reading disability. *In* C. J. Turner and H. B. Miles (eds), *The biology of human intelligence.* Nafferton: Nafferton Books Limited.

Stevenson, J., Graham, P., Fredman, G. and McLoughlin, V. 1987. A twin study of genetic influences on reading and spelling ability and disability. *Journal of Child Psychology and Psychiatry, 28*, 229—247.

Vogel, S. A. 1990. Gender differences in intelligence, language, visual-motor abilities, and academic achievement in males and females with learning disabilities: A review of the literature. *Journal of Learning Disabilities, 23*, 44—52.

Wadsworth, S. J., Gillis, J. J., DeFries, J. C. and Fulker, D. W. 1989. Differential genetic aetiology of reading disability as a function of age. *The Irish Journal of Psychology, 10*, 509—520.

Wechsler, D. 1974. *Examiner's manual: Wechsler Intelligence Scale for Children-Revised.* New York: The Psychological Corporation.

Wechsler, D. 1981. *Examiner's manual: Wechsler Adult Intelligence Scale-Revised.* New York: The Psychological Corporation.

Zerbin-Rüdin, E. 1967. Kongenitale Wortblindheit oder spezifische dyslixie (Congenital Word-Blindness). *Bulletin of the Orton Society, 17*, 47—56.

Screening for Multiple Genes Influencing Dyslexia

SHELLEY D. SMITH[1], WILLIAM J. KIMBERLING[1] and
BRUCE F. PENNINGTON[2]

[1] *Center for Hereditary Communication Disorders, Boys Town National Research Hospital, Omaha, NE;* [2] *University of Denver*

ABSTRACT: Genetic linkage analysis is a means of localizing genes to specific chromosomal regions. Localization of genes influencing specific reading disability (dyslexia) can lead to characterization of the phenotypic effects of each gene and to early diagnosis of children at risk. Previous studies using the family study LOD score method of linkage analysis have identified two chromosomal regions that may contain genes influencing dyslexia. The present study examines the sib pair method of linkage analysis, which has several advantages over the LOD score method. In particular, the mode of inheritance does not need to be specified and diagnosis of parents is not required, but it is a less powerful technique. Using the same population as the previous studies (with less than 200 sib pairs) and two different means of diagnosis of dyslexia, the sib pair analysis was able to detect the same suggested linkages as the LOD score method, plus a possible third region. This confirms that the sib pair method is an effective means of screening for linkage with reasonable sample sizes.

KEYWORDS: dyslexia, genetic linkage, analysis, reading disability, sib pairs.

There are many possible causes of dyslexia, and genes play a role in at least some of these (DeFries, Fulker and LaBuda, 1987). Our goal has been to try to identify one or more of these genes. Once a gene is identified, it can be characterized at a phenotypic and at a molecular level; the phenotype would define what the gene does, and the molecular sequence would tell how it does it. Hopefully, this information would lead to improved remediation at educational or biological levels.

Genes are arrayed linearly along the chromosomes. In humans, there are 23 pairs of homologous chromosomes. One member of each pair is inherited from the mother, and the other from the father. Since chromosomes are in pairs, genes are also in pairs. The two genes in a pair may carry different codes, termed alleles. Since genes are strung together in a specific order on the chromosomes, genes that are close together on the same chromosome tend to be inherited together as the chromosome is transmitted to the offspring. Such genes are said to be linked. However, when homologous chromosomes pair at meiosis, there can be an exchange of DNA between the two chromosomes, which can separate alleles that were previously together. The chance that this recombination will occur is a function of the distance between the two linked loci, such that the

Reading and Writing: An Interdisciplinary Journal 3: 285–298, 1991.
© 1991 *Kluwer Academic Publishers.*

frequency of recombination is a type of measure of the distance between the genes. The chromosomal location of a gene causing a disorder can be found using linkage analysis, which compares the gene's transmission through a family with the transmission of known genetic markers, to determine if the gene and any of the markers are linked.

If the trait dyslexia, for example, is found to be transmitted along with a known marker allele to a statistically significant extent, this is evidence that the dyslexia is influenced by a gene that is close to the marker locus. Once the chromosomal location of a gene is known, molecular methods can be used to find markers that are even closer to the gene, eventually identifying the exact piece of DNA carrying the gene. At that point, the sequence can be determined, which then can lead to identification of the function.

The localization of a gene can also allow determination of genetic heterogeneity; that is, some families may show linkage to one locus, while other families, with a different type of dyslexia, would not show that linkage, but may show linkage to a different locus, implying a different gene which could have a slightly different function. This may result in different phenotypes, or different genes may influence the same basic pathways so that the overall phenotypic effect is very similar. Well characterized families, in which the genetic cause can be documented, would be very valuable for studies into the basic phenotypic defect and the best means of remediation. Also, recognition of the presence of such a gene in a small child would identify him or her as high risk for reading disability and would permit study of precursor deficits and institution of early intervention. (For a more complete description of linkage and its application to reading disability, see Housman, Smith, and Pauls, 1985).

Two methods of linkage analysis have been utilized in the search for genes influencing dyslexia. The first method was the traditional LOD score analysis of extended families (Morton, 1955). Large, three generation, autosomal dominant families were selected for study, and a variety of genetic markers were typed, including blood groups, serum proteins, enzymes, chromosomal heteromorphisms, and DNA restriction fragment length polymorphisms (RFLPs). The transmission of these markers through each family was compared to the transmission of dyslexia using linkage analysis programs LIPED (Ott, 1974) and later LINKAGE (Lathrop et al., 1985). The probability of linkage is expressed as a LOD score, which is an acronym for Log_{10} of the Odds of linkage. The traditional criteria for acceptance of linkage has been a LOD score greater that 3.0, and linkage is rejected if the LOD score is less than −2.0. As more markers have become available for testing, the LOD score criterion for acceptance of linkage will need to be increased, but a general consensus on what this level should be has not been reached.

Initial results indicated a significant linkage with chromosomal heteromorphisms on chromosome 15, with a recombination fraction of about 30% (Smith et al., 1983). However, with the addition of more families, the evidence for linkage decreased in some of the families, but not in all. One family in particular maintained a very high LOD score, which is currently at 2.9 with no recombination. This led to the suspicion that there could be genetic heterogeneity, that is, more than one gene that could produce dyslexia. A statistical test of heterogeneity was done using the program HOMOG (Ott, 1985), and this confirmed that, if there is linkage, only about 20% of the 22 families were linked to chromosome 15, with a recombination fraction of zero (Smith et al., 1990).

With this evidence for heterogeneity, the data were examined for evidence of another locus that might be linked. Suggestive LOD scores were noted for markers on chromosome 6, and further typing was done on that chromosome. Although not significant, the results were quite intriguing, for several reasons. First of all, the LOD scores for chromosome 6 markers BF and GLO showed heterogeneity, with about 20% of families linked when the entire population of 22 families was considered. Furthermore, families who showed positive linkage with chromosome 15 tended to show negative scores with chromosome 6 and vice versa (Smith el al., 1989; DeFries et al., 1990). In fact, when the one family (6432) which showed very high probability of linkage with 15 was omitted from the analysis for chromosome 6 markers, the linkage became statistically significant ($p < 0.001$) under the hypothesis that about 80% of families were linked.

There are several limitations to the extended family study LOD score method of analysis. First of all, these analyses were done assuming autosomal dominant genes with complete penetrance in males and females. Segregation analysis of these families, however, indicated decreased penetrance in females (Pennington et al., in review). These estimates of penetrance can be inserted in the linkage analysis. This relates to the more serious concern, which is that the family study method requires that a diagnosis, whether qualitative or quantitative, be applied to each family member. Not only does this mean that extended families over several generations should be examined, which can be logistically difficult, but it means that accurate diagnosis is needed across a wide range of ages. Diagnosis of reading disability can be very difficult in adults who may have compensated for an earlier reading disability, and thus would not show clear deficits on testing. Finally, there may be genes with other modes of inheritance that were not detected by the family study method when an autosomal dominant mode of inheritance was assumed.

Another method for linkage analysis is the sib pair method. In contrast to the family study method, it does not require assumptions about penetrance nor mode of inheritance, and the diagnosis is specified only for the siblings being studied, allowing the age range to be restricted if necessary. The disadvantage of the sib pair technique is that it is less powerful than the family study method and may require many more individuals for analysis, particularly if the marker locus is not tightly linked. Still, it is a good technique for screening for genes that may contribute to a complex trait.

The principle behind sib pair analysis is that siblings who are concordant for genes influencing dyslexia will be concordant for closely linked genes as well, and sibs that are discordant for dyslexia will be discordant for the linked genes (Haseman and Elston, 1972). Thus, the analysis is based only on pairs of sibs, and the mode of inheritance and the diagnosis of their parents is unimportant. However, the *marker* genotypes of the parents can be important, since this will indicate whether or not the siblings are segregating for a given marker. If the parents are both homozygous for an allele, the fact that their two affected children are both concordant for the marker allele is meaningless. The method depends upon being able to tell if the shared alleles are "identical by descent" (ibd), that is, that alleles that the sibs share were inherited from the same parent and thus are accompanied by the same linked alleles. A pair of siblings can be identical by descent for 0, 1, or 2 alleles. For some matings, this will be quite clear; if the parents have 4 different alleles, it is clear which allele in the offspring came from which parent, and the association with the trait is unambiguous. However, sometimes the parental origin of an allele cannot be determined reliably, and an estimate of the alleles identical by descent must be made. The sib pair method we are using is based on the Haseman and Elston (1972) method for searching for loci that contribute to a quantitative trait, although a qualitative diagnosis can also be used. Basically, the trait variables are figures for a pair of sibs, and the squared difference between their scores is regressed upon their proportion of alleles identical by descent for a given locus. If the alleles at that locus are linked to the alleles influencing the trait measure, there will be a significant linear relationship between them, such that a small difference between sibs in the trait variable should be associated with a high probability of identity by descent, and a larger difference in the trait measure should be associated with low ibd values.

As with the family study method, sib pair linkage analysis will be thwarted by genetic heterogeneity. One way to allow for this is to subdivide the population based on predetermined clinical criteria and see if different linkages are detected in different subgroups. The danger is that the sample size will be too small to detect a real linkage.

METHODOLOGY

Marker data were obtained from 18 families which had been ascertained for our previous studies. Details of their selection have been reported elsewhere (Smith et al., 1983). In these families, the transmission of dyslexia is consistent with an autosomal dominant mode of inheritance. The Sibpal program of the SAGE package developed by Elston and colleagues (Tran et al., 1989) was utilized for the sib pair analyses. This utilizes the Haseman-Elston algorithm described above, in which the number of alleles ibd is regressed on the trait measure; in this case, the diagnosis.

Two different diagnostic criteria were utilized in the sib pair analyses. First, the diagnosis was specified as a qualitative trait. Sibs were either diagnosed as affected or unaffected, according to a paradigm developed in conjunction with Dr. Bruce Pennington (Pennington et al., 1984). The analyses were also done using a quantitative measure of dyslexia, the discriminant score developed by DeFries et al. (1987). Since this population was originally selected for family studies, it includes adult siblings, so there may be some loss of information if the discriminant score, which is based on current test results, is not sensitive to compensation. Still, it could be that compensated adults would be more like their compensated sibs than their normal sibs, so that there could still be some differentiation between "concordant" and "discordant" sibs. Discriminant scores were not available for all of the family members, so the population is slightly smaller.

Loci from the two chromosomal regions suggested by our previous studies were analysed. The markers for chromosome 15 are shown in Figure 1. All of the markers are RFLP's except for the cen15 marker, which is the centromeric and short arm cytogenetic heteromorphism.

Four chromosome 6 markers, BF, GLO, thh157, and 2C5 were included. BF (properdin factor) is a serum protein, GLO (Glyoxylase 1) is a red cell enzyme, and thh157 and 2C5 are RFLPs. They are located on the short arm of chromosome 6, bands p21.31—p21.1. The HLA loci are also in the region of 6p21.3, and GLO is about 3 cM distal to the HLA loci (McKusick, 1990).

Because of the evidence for heterogeneity in this population, the data were also analysed with and without family 6432, the family which showed very significant linkage to the chromosome 15 heteromorphism marker by the LOD score method. This family contained 24 sib pairs.

RESULTS

Qualitative Diagnosis

Chromosome 15

Table 1 shows the number of siblings for which marker data were available for each marker, and Table 2 gives the results of the regression analysis.

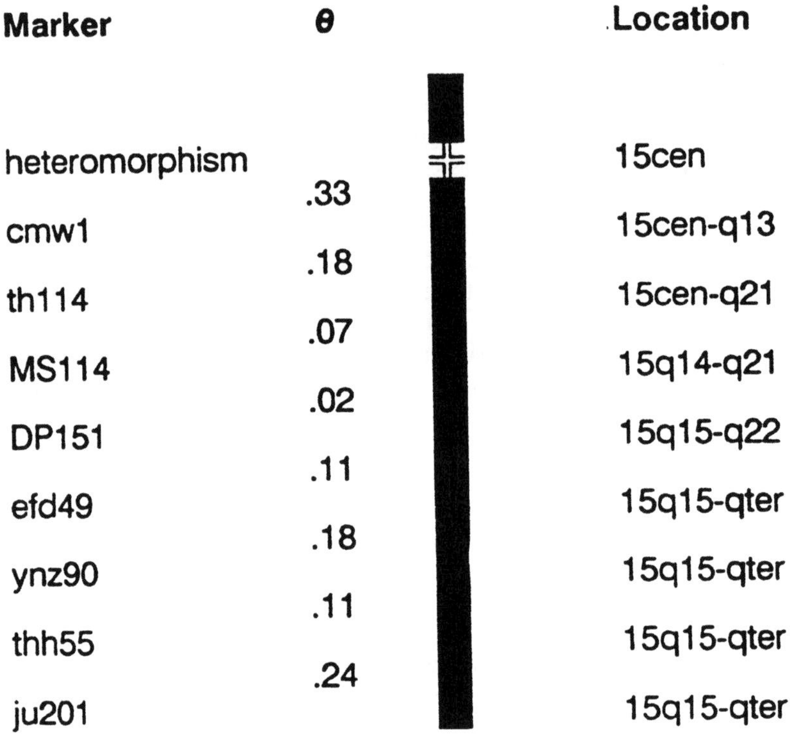

Fig. 1. Relative Position of Chrosome 15 markers.

The results showed significant regression of the trait with one marker, ynz90. As can be seen in Figure 1, this marker is not near the centromere, where the initial linkage was found, and was not significant in the LOD score analysis. It may be a spurious linkage or it may indicate a locus that is not dominantly inherited, so that it would have been missed in the LOD score analysis. Certainly, it will be important to see if this result is replicated in a separate population.

When only family 6432 was considered in the sib pair analysis, the results for the centromeric heteromorphisms were significant at the 0.05 level (Table 3). This is less significant that the LOD score analysis, which takes into account all of the family members and transmission between them, but still indicates that, when there is tight linkage, a significant indication of linkage can still be detected in a small set of sibs.

Table 1. Sib Pair Analysis with Chromosome 15 Markers

marker	Number of pairs concordant unaffected	discordant	concordant affected	total
cen 15	9	55	91	155
cmwl	8	61	103	172
th114	5	13	35	53
pDP151	10	61	100	171
pMS114	10	60	99	169
ynz90	5	32	74	111
thh55	4	22	28	54
ju201	7	56	98	161

Table 2. Sib Pair Analysis with Chromosome 15 Markers

	Qualitative trait simple regression analysis		
marker	df	*t*-values	*p*-values
cen15	153	−0.7896	0.2155
cmwl	170	−0.0525	0.4791
th114	51	−0.3360	0.3691
pDP151	169	1.2380	0.8913
pMS114	167	0.5928	0.7320
ynz90	109	−2.4236	0.0085**
thh55	52	−0.7380	0.2319
ju201	159	0.7262	0.7656

Table 3. Sib Pair Analysis with Chromosome 15 Markers, Family 6432 Only

	Qualitative trait simple regression analysis		
marker	df	*t*-values	*p*-values
cen15	22	−2.0164	0.0281*
cmw1	13	1.1154	0.8576
pDP151	15	1.0526	0.8454
pMS114	15	1.1337	0.8626
ju201	13	1.4619	0.9162

Chromosome 6

The number of siblings with marker typing are shown in Table 4, and the results of the analysis are given in Table 5. The marker GLO showed significance at the 0.05 level.

Again, because of its significant linkage with chromosome 15, family 6432 was omitted to see if this had an effect on the linkage with chromosome 6 markers. Even with the decreased sample size, the significance of the regression increased to the 0.01 level, indicating that family 6432 was contributing negative data (Table 6). This can be seen graphically in Figure 2, which shows the regression lines obtained by the entire population and by the population with family 6432 omitted.

Table 4. Sib Pair Analysis with Chromosome 6 Markers

	Number of pairs			
marker	concordant unaffected	discordant	concordant affected	total
BF	10	61	104	175
thh157	6	52	97	155
2C5	7	47	86	140
GLO	10	61	101	172

Table 5. Sib Pair Analysis with Chromosome 6 Markers

	Qualitative trait simple regression analysis		
marker	df	*t*-values	*p*-values
BF	173	−1.1708	0.1217
thh157	153	0.5701	0.7153
2C5	138	−1.6021	0.0557
GLO	170	−2.1795	0.0153*

Quantitative Diagnosis

Chromosome 15

The results of the sib pair analysis with chromosome 15 markers gave no evidence of linkage with chromosome 15 heteromorphisms when the

Table 6. Sib Pair Analysis with Chromosome 6 Markers, Omitting Family 6432

	Qualitative trait simple regression analysis		
marker	df	*t*-values	*p*-values
BF	156	−1.3750	0.0856
thh157	140	0.8291	0.7958
2C5	124	−1.3167	0.0952
GLO	153	−2.3931	0.0090**

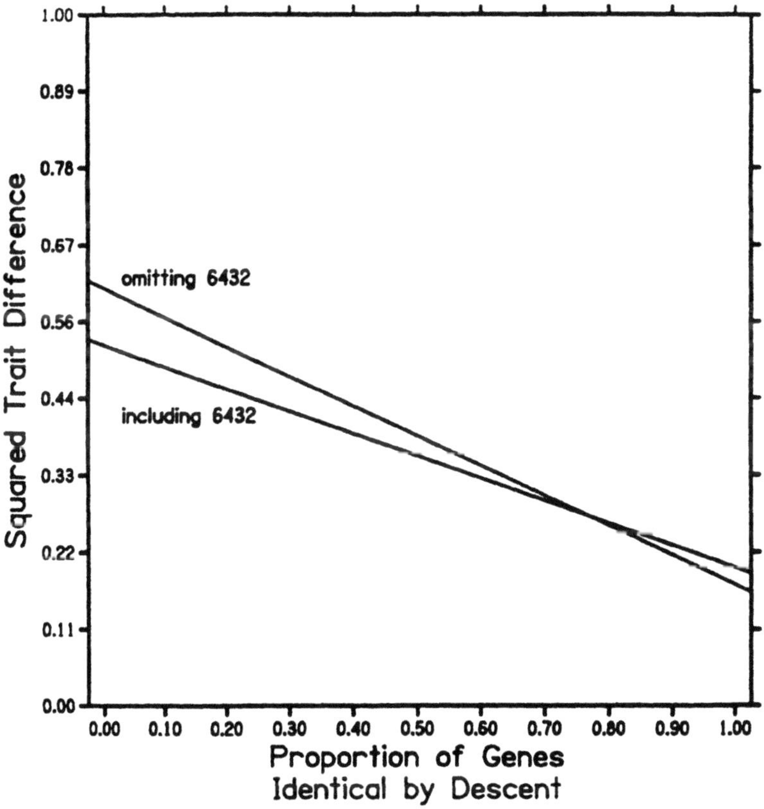

Fig. 2. Squared Trait Differences OF RD Vs. The Proportion Of Genes IBD At Locus GLO With and Without Family 6432.

population as a whole was considered (Table 7), but again there is slight significance for a marker farther down the chromosome arm. Marker ju201, which is significant at the 0.05 level, is located in the same region ynz90.

When only family 6432 was analysed, there was no significance for the chromosome 15 heteromorphisms nor ju201 (Table 8). This family contains a number of compensated women, so it may be that the discriminant score is not sensitive enough to compensation. It is also possible that the phenotype in this family is slightly different, such that the discriminant score is not as good a measure of the gene effect. Finally, it is possible that the linkage to ju201 is looser and a larger sample size is required to detect it.

Table 7. Sib Pair Analysis with Chromosome 15 Markers

	Qualitative trait simple regression analysis		
marker	df	*t*-values	*p*-values
cen15	130	−0.9501	0.1719
cmwl	140	−1.2355	0.8907
th114	39	2.3295	0.9874
pDP151	141	1.0099	0.8429
pMS114	139	−0.6701	0.2519
ynz90	81	−1.4876	0.0704
thh55	43	0.8866	0.8099
ju201	130	−1.8397	0.0340*

Table 8. Sib Pair Analysis with Chromosome 15 Markers, Family 6432 Only

	Qualitative trait simple regression analysis		
marker	df	*t*-values	*p*-values
cen15	15	−1.4019	0.0931
cmwl	10	−0.4006	0.3486
pDP151	12	1.3285	0.8956
pMS114	12	0.8506	0.7942
ju201	10	−1.1864	0.4279

Chromosome 6

The results of the sib pair analysis using the quantitative trait measure produced comparable results for the chromosome 6 markers (Table 9). The marker BF rather than GLO was significant; since these loci are linked, this probably reflects a difference in diagnosis that affects the recombination fraction, but the same region is still indicated. This time, however, the significance is greater than the 0.001 level, which could be considered equivalent to a LOD score greater than 3. The regression line is shown in Figure 3.

Omission of family 6432 from the analysis gave essentially the same highly significant results for BF, and 2C5 also showed some significance (Table 10). This marker is located between BF and GLO. Again, this may reflect the presence of a gene in this region, with the different diagnostic criteria and different population subsets affecting the recombination detected between specific loci. The significance level is actually greater for the discriminant measure than for the dichotomous diagnosis, which could mean that the discriminant score is a better measure of this phenotype (as opposed to the phenotype in families that do not show linkage to chromo-

Table 9. Sib Pair Analysis with Chromosome 6 Markers

	Qualitative trait simple regression analysis		
marker	df	*t*-values	*p*-values
BF	142	−4.1364	0.0000***
thh157	125	−1.3139	0.0956
2C5	121	−1.5726	0.0592
GLO	144	−0.7336	0.2322

Table 10. Sib Pair Analysis with Chromosome 6 Markers, Omitting Family 6432

	Qualitative trait simple regression analysis		
marker	df	*t*-values	*p*-values
BF	128	−3.7819	0.0001***
thh157	113	−0.8315	0.2037
2C5	110	−1.9361	0.0277*
GLO	130	−1.0243	0.1538

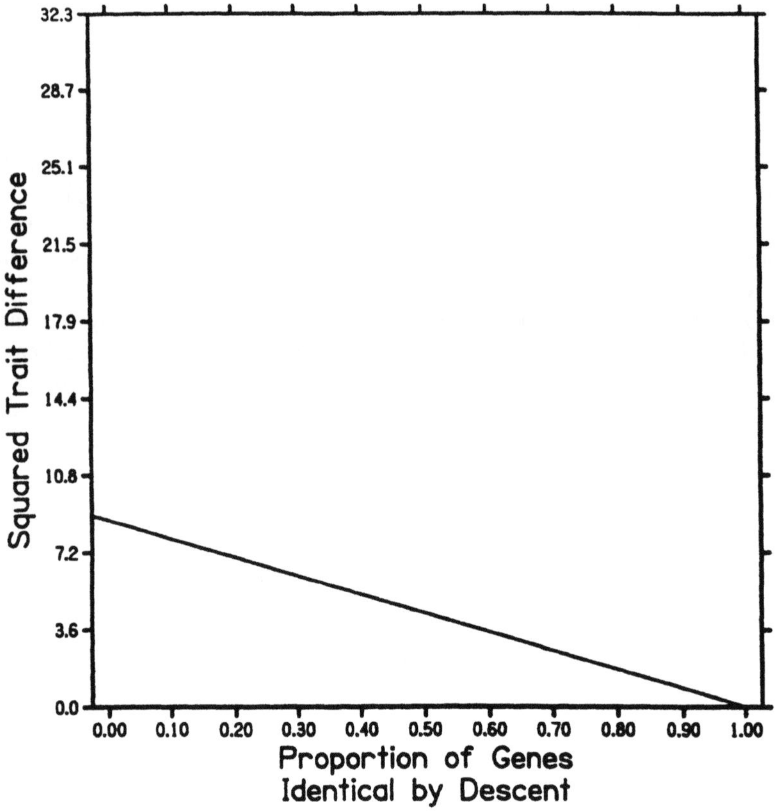

Fig. 3. Squared Quantitative Trait Differences Of RD Vs. the Proportion Of Genes IBD At Locus BF.

some 6). If the putative gene on chromosome 6 accounts for a larger proportion of the population (as suggested by the homogeneity analysis of the LOD score data), it is possible that more of the individuals in the population from which the discriminant function was derived had this form of dyslexia. It could even indicate that the discriminant function is picking up a subtle deficit in individuals which the dichotomous method called "normal" (and thus would have represented a cross-over in the previous analyses).

CONCLUSION

All together, these studies show that the sib pair method can be used to screen for loci that may or may not be dominant; further studies with an expanded population will show whether these significance levels are confirmed. The family studies, using an autosomal dominant hypothesis, can be used to determine if any markers so identified are also seen with that method. So far, it can be concluded that there may be a locus on chromosome 6 which has a major effect on dyslexia; that there may be another, rarer gene near the centromeric region of 15 that has a major effect; and that there may even be a non-dominant gene farther down on the long arm of 15. Further studies will show if these can be confirmed in a separate population. The slightly different results seen with the two diagnostic methods demonstrates that diagnosis is critical to linkage analysis, and that an even more sensitive criteria, such as a measure of phonological coding, may improve the ability to detect linkage.

AUTHORS NOTES

This work was supported by NIH grant PO1 HD11681, by NIMH grants M419 (RJDA to BFP) and MH38820, and by a March of Dimes Grant 12—135. Some of the results reported in this paper were obtained by using the program package S.A.G.E., which is supported by U.S. Public Health Service resource grant RR03655 from the Division of Research Resources. Reprints may be requested from S. D. Smith, Boys Town National Institute, 555 N. 30th St., Omaha, NE 68131.

REFERENCES

DeFries, J. C., Fulker, D. W., and LaBuda, M. C. 1987. Evidence for a genetic aetiology in reading disability of twins. *Nature, 329*, 537—539.

DeFries, J. C., Olson, R. C., Pennington, B. F., and Smith, S. D. 1991 Colorado Reading Project: An Update. In Gray, D., and Duane, D. (Eds.), *The reading brain: The biological basis of dyslexia*. Parkton, MD: York Press

Haseman, J. K. and Elston, R. C. 1972. The investigation of linkage between a quantitative trait and a marker locus. *Behavior Genetics, 2*, 3—19.

Housman, D., Smith, S. D., and Pauls, D. 1985. Applications of Recombinant DNA to Neurogenetic Disorders. In Gray, D. B. and Kavanagh, J. F. (Eds.), *Biobehavioral Measures of Dyslexia* (pp. 155—162). Parkton, MD: York Press.

Lathrop, G. M., Lalouel, J. M., Julier, C., and Ott, J. 1985. Multilocus linkage analysis in humans: Detection of linkage and estimation of recombination. *American Journal of Human Genetics, 37*, 482—498.

McKusick, V. A. 1990. *Mendelian Inheritance in Man: Catalogs of Autosomal Dominant, Autosomal Recessive, and X-Linked Phenotypes, Ninth Edition*. Baltimore: The Johns Hopkins University Press.

Morton, N. E. 1955. Sequential tests for the detection of linkage. *American Journal of Human Genetics, 7*, 277—328.

Ott, J. 1974. Estimation of the recombination fraction in human pedigrees: Efficient computation of the likelihood for human studies. *American Journal of Human Genetics, 26*, 588–597.

Ott, J. 1985. *Analysis of human genetic linkage*. Baltimore: The Johns Hopkins University Press.

Pennington, B. F., Gilgler, J., Pauls, D., Smıth, S. A., Smith, S. D., and DeFries, J. C. (in review). Evidence for a major gene transmission of developmental dyslexia.

Pennington, B. F., Smith, S. D., McCabe, L. L., Kimberling, W. J., and Lubs, H. A. 1984. Development continuities and discontinuities in a form of familial dyslexia. *In* Emde, R. and Harman, R. (Eds.), *Continuities and Discontinuities in Development* (pp. 123–151). New York: Plenum.

Smith, S. D., Kimberling, W. J., Pennington, B. F., and Lubs, H. A. 1983. Specific reading disability: Identification of an inherited form through linkage analysis. *Science, 219*, 1345–1347.

Smith, S. D., Kimberling, W. J., Shugart, Y. Y., Ing, P. S., and Pennington, B. F. 1989. Genetic linkage analysis of 20 families with specific reading disability, *American Journal of Human Genetics, 45*, A65. Presented to the American Society of Human Genetics, Baltimore, November 12, 1989.

Smith, S. D., Pennington, B. F., Kimberling, W. J., and Ing, P. S. 1990. Familial dyslexia: Use of genetic linkage data to define subtypes. *Journal of the American Academy of Child and Adolescent Psychiatry, 29*, 204–213.

Tran, L. D., Elston, R. C., Keats, B. J. B., and Wilson, A. F. 1989. Sib-Pair linkage program (SIBPAL) User's Guide. Part of the S.A.G.E. 89 Release 2.0 documentation, University of Louisiana Medical Center, New Orleans, LA.

Multiple Regression Analysis of Sib-Pair Data on Reading to Detect Quantitative Trait Loci

D. W. FULKER,[1] L. R. CARDON,[1] J. C. DEFRIES,[1]
W. J. KIMBERLING,[3] B. F. PENNINGTON [2] and S. D. SMITH[3]

[1] *Institute for Behavioral Genetics, University of Colorado, Boulder, CO 80309* [2] *Department of Psychology, University of Denver, Denver, CO 80208* [3] *Boys Town National Institute for Communication Disorders in Children, Omaha, NE 68010*

ABSTRACT: A simple extension of the DeFries and Fulker multiple regression model for twin analysis is applied to the problem of detecting linkage in a quantitative trait. The method, employing sib pairs, is based on that of Haseman and Elston. Reading data from 19 extended pedigrees were analyzed employing RLFPs as markers on chromosome 15 and using the widely available statistical applications software package, SAS. A number of possible linkages were detected, indicating that this approach is both powerful and effective, especially in the case of selected samples. Detecting genotype—environment interaction and the issue of power are briefly discussed. The programs used are available upon request.

KEYWORDS: multiple regression, quantitative trait loci, sib-pair data, reading disability, linkage analysis.

INTRODUCTION

This paper describes a simple application of the DeFries and Fulker (1985, 1988) multiple regression analysis of twin data to the problem of detecting linkage in a quantitative trait. It combines the regression approach with that of Haseman and Elston (1972), which uses sibling data on the trait together with information on identity by descent (ibd) for marker loci to which the quantitative trait loci (QTLs) may be genetically linked. While the approach we suggest is not a radical departure from that of Haseman and Elston, we believe it offers a number of advantages over their approach.

Firstly, our approach is conceptually very straightforward. Secondly, it is simple to apply, only requiring one of the widely used statistical packages such as SAS or SPSS. Thirdly, it is equally applicable to selected samples as well as unselected samples, providing a simple unified approach to sibling linkage analysis. Fourthly, it is very flexible, permitting the evaluation of variables that may interact with QTL genotypic effects such as sex or age. And fifthly, it appears to be more statistically powerful than the standard Haseman and Elston approach, particularly when applied to selected samples.

Reading and Writing: An Interdisciplinary Journal **3**: 299—313, 1991.
© 1991 *Kluwer Academic Publishers.*

While other approaches may be more appropriate in some specific situations we believe the features listed above make the regression approach extremely useful for those who need a simple straightforward method for detecting polygenes or QTLs in order to undertake exploratory data analysis or rapid screening of genetic markers.

In this paper the method is outlined and then illustrated using sibling data on reading performance as a quantitative trait and restriction fragment length polymorphisms (RFLPs) on chromosome 15 as genetic markers.

REGRESSION MODEL

The regression approach to the analysis of twin data exists in two forms, one employing the basic model and the other the augmented model. The basic model is intended for use with selected samples and involves the idea that differential regression to the population mean of MZ and DZ cotwins of selected probands indicates the presence of heritable variation. The cotwin score on a quantitative trait (C) is entered into the analysis as the dependent variable in a regression equation with the proband score (P) and the coefficient of relationship (R), which takes values 1.0 for MZ pairs and 1/2 for DZ pairs, entered as independent variables. The regression equation, including the constant term A, is given below.

$$C = B_1 P + B_2 R + A \tag{1}$$

The B_1 regression weight adjusts the cotwin score for average twin resemblance while the B_2 term measures the extent of differential regression of cotwins' means back towards the mean of the population. A significant B_2 term indicates the presence of a heritable component in the proband mean. The method has the advantage of increasing statistical power as a function of the degree of selection imposed on the probands, thus requiring fewer and fewer twin pairs the more intense the selection becomes.

The underlying principle of the method may be seen in Figure 1, in which the distribution at the top of the figure represents that of the base population with a selected group of low scoring individuals at the tail of the distribution labeled probands. The distributions of the MZ and DZ cotwins are shown below and can be seen to have means regressing back towards that of the population, μ, but more so for DZ than for MZ pairs. It can be shown (DeFries and Fulker, 1988) that B_1 is an estimate of the average twin correlation and that $B_2 = 2[(\overline{C}_{MZ} - \overline{C}_{DZ}) - B_1 (\overline{P}_M - \overline{P}_{DZ})]$ or just $2(\overline{C}_{MZ} - \overline{C}_{DZ})$ when the two kinds of probands have the same mean, which is usually expected to be the case. This regression coefficient, when divided by the selection differential, $\overline{P} - \mu$, is an estimate of the herit-

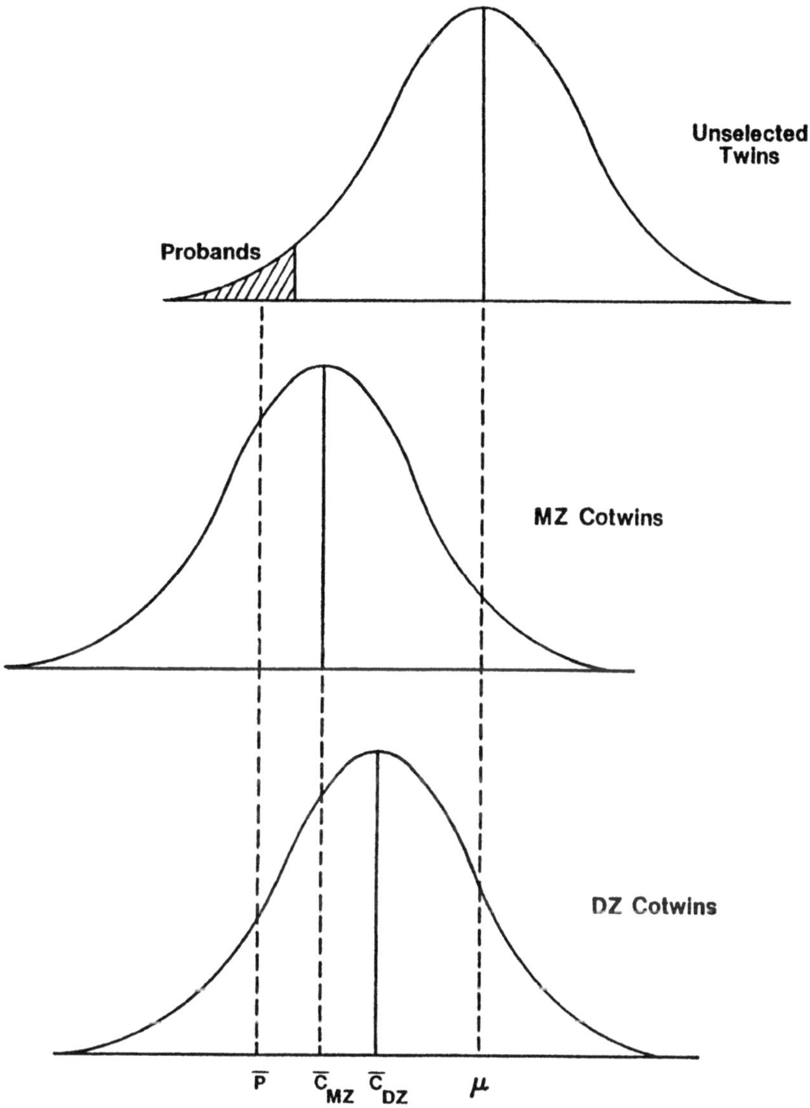

Fig. 1. Hypothetical distributions for reading performance of an unselected sample of twins and of the identical (MZ) and fraternal (DZ) cotwins of probands with a reading disability. The differential regression of the MZ and DZ cotwin means toward the mean of the unselected population (μ) provides a test of genetic etiology. [From DeFries, Fulker, and LaBuda (1987). Reprinted by permission from *Nature*, Vol. 329, p. 537. Copyright © 1987, Macmillan Magazines Ltd.]

ability of the proband deficit, h_g^2. If this deficit is due to the same factors that cause individual differences in the general population, then it is also an estimate of heritability (h^2) in the population as a whole.

In the augmented model a fourth term, PR, the product of proband score and the coefficient of relationship, is added to equation (1) to give (2).

$$C = B_3P + B_4R + B_5PR + A \quad (2)$$

In this form the coefficient B_5 is a direct estimate of h^2 and B_3 is a direct estimate of shared environmental variance c^2. When scores are expressed as deviations from the population mean (μ) and divided by $\overline{P} - \mu$, the coefficient B_4 estimates $h_g^2 - h^2$. The addition of the product PR assesses differential twin resemblances as a function of zygosity, which is the basis for inferring h^2 from the twin design and is no more than $2(B_{MZ} - B_{DZ})$, or $2(R_{MZ} - R_{DZ})$, where B and R are simple twin regressions and correlations calculated from a random sample of twins, which is a standard way to estimate h^2.

The advantages of the regression method over the evaluation of correlations is its convenience for those not familiar with model fitting procedures, its flexibility for testing for interactions with other variable such as gender (Cyphers et al., 1990), and the fact that by using regression rather than correlations a correction for selection on the probands is applied. Thus, the augmented model is applicable to the analysis of continuous variation in both unselected and selected samples.

HASEMAN AND ELSTON LINKAGE MODEL

The Haseman and Elston (1972) approach to linkage uses information on marker loci in siblings and their parents to determine the proportion of alleles two siblings share ibd. This number, which they call π, can only take values zero, one half, or one, corresponding to ibd status zero, one, and two, and indicates how closely the pair resemble each other genetically at this locus. With a value of zero siblings are no more alike than totally unrelated individuals, with a value of one half they are as alike as ordinary siblings are on average for any locus, and with a value of one they are identical just like identical twins.

Thus, if a QTL is at that locus or closely linked to it, the three kinds of siblings should show differential resemblance, those with π equal to one being more alike than those with π equal to one half, who in turn should be more alike than those pairs with π equal to zero. Haseman and Elston use the sib pair difference squared (Y) as a measure of resemblance. Since this is technically twice the within pair variance for each pair of sibs, the three values of π should relate inversely to this measure of resemblance if there is any linkage. Consequently the regression of Y on π is expected to be negative if the marker is near a QTL influencing the phenotype. They show that the regression coefficient will be equal to the additive genetic variance of the QTL multiplied by $-2(1 - 2\theta)^2$, where θ is the recombination fraction between the marker locus and the QTL ($0 \leqslant \theta \leqslant 0.5$). Therefore, when θ is zero the regression will detect all the genetic variance due to the QTL; however, when θ is as much as 0.12, or approximately twelve centimorgans away from the marker, only half the genetic variance of the QTL will be detected.

The ideal situation for the application of their approach is when the marker locus is completely informative regarding the ibd status of the sibs. For two allele markers, which are the most common, this is seldom the case and the method was initially criticized on these grounds (Robertson, 1973). However, with the advent of more recent molecular markers, which are increasingly polymorphic, the method has become much more promising. Nance and Neale (1989), who recently modified the Haseman and Elston approach for use with twin data using LISREL, illustrate this fact with a table of parental genotypes involving a four allele system in which the parents are both heterozygous for different alleles. That is, one parent is A_1A_2 and the other A_3A_4. Under these conditions ibd status is clearly unambiguous since it is obvious from which parent the alleles came and whether or not they are the same. Table 1, modified from their paper, illustrates the point.

However, not all markers are so informative; indeed, some are totally uninformative and Haseman and Elston introduced an ingenious refinement into their method to account for such markers. When they cannot

Table 1. Number of Alleles ibd for Marker Locus

Parents' Genotypes
$A_1A_2 \times A_3A_4$

		Sib 1			
		A_1A_3	A_2A_3	A_1A_4	A_2A_4
Sib 2	A_1A_3	2	1	1	0
	A_2A_3	1	2	0	1
	A_1A_4	1	0	2	1
	A_2A_4	0	1	1	2

# IBD	π
0	0
1	1/2
2	1

determine π unambiguously from the markers, they estimate it ($\hat{\pi}$) instead. The method is shown in Table 2 taken from their paper and it involves forming a weighted average of the probabilities that 0, 1, or 2 sibling alleles are identical by descent given both sibling and the parental genotypes. These probabilities they denote as f_{j0}, f_{j1}, and f_{j2}, respectively, for the jth locus. The estimate of $\hat{\pi}$ is then simply $1/2f_{j1} + f_{j2}$. It can be seen from the table that the estimates ($\hat{\pi}$) are the same as π when sufficiently informative markers are available, as in those cases where only one value of f_j appears in any given row. From this table any value of $\hat{\pi}$ can be obtained by simply locating the appropriate combination of parental and sibling genotypes from among the 34 possibilities. The original paper proves that $\hat{\pi}$ provides an unbiased estimate of π. The computer program SIBPAL carries out the Haseman and Elston analysis and is available commercially.

COMBINED MODEL

The essence of the approach we suggest is simply to replace the coefficient of relationship in the DeFries and Fulker regression approach with the

Table 2. $\hat{\pi}_j$ When Both Parental and Sib Genotypes Are Known

Mating type	Sib-pair type	f_{j0}	f_{j1}	f_{j2}	$\hat{\pi}_j$
I: $A_iA_i \times A_iA_i$	I: $A_iA_i - A_iA_i$	¼	½	¼	½
II: $A_iA_i \times A_jA_j$	V: $A_iA_j - A_iA_j$	¼	½	¼	½
III: $A_iA_i \times A_iA_j$	I: $A_iA_i - A_iA_i$	0	½	½	¾
	III: $A_iA_i - A_iA_j$	½	½	0	¼
	V: $A_iA_j - A_iA_j$	0	½	½	¾
IV: $A_iA_i \times A_jA_k$	V: (2)	0	½	½	¾
	VI: $A_iA_j - A_iA_k$	½	½	0	¼
V: $A_iA_j \times A_iA_j$	I: (2)	0	0	1	1
	II: $A_iA_i - A_jA_j$	1	0	0	0
	III: (2)	0	1	0	½
	V: $A_iA_j - A_iA_j$	½	0	½	½
VI: $A_iA_j \times A_iA_k$	I: $A_iA_i - A_iA_i$	0	0	1	1
	III: (2)	0	1	0	½
	IV: $A_iA_i - A_jA_k$	1	0	0	0
	V: (3)	0	0	1	1
	VI: $A_iA_j - A_iA_k$	1	0	0	0
	VI: $A_iA_j - A_jA_k$	0	1	0	½
	VI: $A_iA_k - A_jA_k$	0	1	0	½
VII: $A_iA_j \times A_kA_l$	V: (4)	0	0	1	1
	VI: (4)	0	1	0	½
	VII: (2)	1	0	0	0

value of $\hat{\pi}$, and employ data on pairs of sibs in the place of those on twins. Thus, the basic model becomes

$$C = B_1P + B_2\hat{\pi} + A \quad (3)$$

and the augmented model becomes

$$C = B_3P + B_4\hat{\pi} + B_5P\hat{\pi} + A \quad (4)$$

Since $\hat{\pi}$ performs the same function as R in modelling sib resemblance in terms of additive genetic variance — not of the whole genome but for the QTL associated with specific marker locus in question — the regression coefficients B_2 and B_5 test for h_g^2 and h^2 of the QTL when the linkage is complete. When the QTL is θ centimorgans from the marker, these heritabilities are reduced by a factor $(1 - 2\theta)^2$, as shown in Haseman and Elston's paper.

The coefficient B_1 in the basic model provides a measure of average sib resemblance. However, B_3 in the augmented model assesses the average sib resemblance due to all sources of variation, both genetic and environmental, other than that due to the QTL. Since this resemblance is often substantial, the control for this source of variation in the regression approach should add power to that of Haseman and Elston.

Although the sample size in the present analysis is not sufficient to allow tests of gender X genotype interaction, it is of interest to show how simple it is to incorporate interactions into the model. If the main effect of gender (or any other main effect such as remediation) is designated S and introduced into the basic model, then three more regression coefficients are required.

$$C = B_1P + B_2\hat{\pi} + B_{10}S + B_{11}SP + B_{12}S\hat{\pi} + A \quad (5)$$

In the augmented model four more regression coefficients are required.

$$C = B_3P + B_4\hat{\pi} + B_5P\hat{\pi} + B_6S + B_7SP + B_8S\hat{\pi} + B_9SP\hat{\pi} + A \quad (6)$$

The terms B_{12} in the basic model and B_9 in the augmented model test for genotype X gender interaction.

METHODS

Subjects

The subjects used to illustrate the method are members of 19 three-generation families with a history of reading disability that have been the subject of a series of linkage studies which started with nine families and a chromosomal marker on 15 (Smith et al., 1983). Since that time families have been added to the study and 9 RFLP markers have been typed on chromosome 15. A recent update on the Colorado Reading Study provides a summary of research methods and findings (DeFries et al., 1991). For the present purpose it is sufficient to note that a variety of analyses have indicated linkage to the disorder on chromosome 15 and familial heterogeneity. The subjects are those used by Smith et al. in the present volume.

These 19 families yield 161 sib pairs for analysis. Although the pairs are not all independent of each other when formed in this way, it appears that the assumption of independence is not important (Blackwelder and Elston, 1985). In order to label one sib a proband and the other a cosib, we employed two procedures depending on whether selection was used or not. With no selection all pairs were double entered and standard errors of the regression weights adjusted by a factor of the square root of two, a procedure routinely applied in the regression procedure when used with pairs of twins. In the case of subsets of the sibs selected for extreme scores all pairs were again double entered before selection in order to allow either sib to be a proband if he or she met the selection criterion. Then standard errors were rescaled, this time by the square root of the ratio of the total number of pairs entered into the analysis to that number minus the number of double entered pairs. These procedures take account of the method of ascertainment and the statistical problems associated with double entry (DeFries et al., 1991).

Test Scores

The subjects have been evaluated in a variety of ways. However, for the present analysis a discriminant score based on the Peabody Individual Achievement Test (PIAT; Dunn and Markwardt, 1970) Reading Recognition, Reading Comprehension and Spelling scores of the sibs was used. Details of how the discriminant score was constructed are given by DeFries (1985). Typical z scores range from about plus two to minus five with those in the present sample being low due to the initial identification of families with reading problems.

Markers

The 9 markers on chromosome 15 used in the present analysis are all RFLPs typed in the laboratory of Drs. Smith and Kimberling. They are shown in Table 3 in the results section. A more detailed description is given in Smith et al. in the present volume.

Analysis

The analysis was conducted using the models described above and a SAS program (SAS Institute, 1988) that read in data in the standard pedigree format employed by the program SIBPAL, sorted subjects into sib pairs, carried out the required degree of phenotypic selection for the purpose of comparisons of power and input the data into the regression routine of SAS. Where marker information was not sufficient to estimate $\hat{\pi}$ using Table 2, we omitted the sib pair from the analysis. Haseman and Elston provide a more elegant solution to this problem, but we chose to take the present more conservative approach. These programs were written by the second author (LRC) to run on mainframe or personal computers and are available on one diskette with explanatory notes, free of charge, upon request.

It should be noted that the sorting of the data into pairs and calculation of the $\hat{\pi}$s is the major task performed by SAS. Once these tasks have been performed the regression analysis can be undertaken using any simple statistical package on a PC or indeed using a pocket calculator.[1]

RESULTS

Univariate Analyses

Five analyses were carried out for each of the 9 markers. The first was a direct application of the Haseman and Elston approach, but using our own program, and was employed as a comparison with our own approach. The second was an application of the DeFries and Fulker augmented model, which differs from the Haseman and Elston approach only insofar that the average sib resemblance is controlled for in the analysis, presumably increasing power. The remaining three analyses involved the basic model applied to probands selected for a phenotypic score of less than 0, −1, and −2, respectively. The results of these analyses are given in Table 3, in the form of *t*-tests (adjusted for double entry) of the significance of β for the Haseman and Elston analysis, B_5 in the case of the augmented DeFries and Fulker model and B_2 in the case of the basic model.

The Haseman and Elston analysis given in the first row of Table 3 detects a significant effect for the marker ju201 at the end of the long arm. The same result was obtained using SIBPAL (Smith et al., this volume). The augmented DeFries and Fulker model detects the same effect. In addition, however, one other locus is detected, ynz90. When selection is imposed and the basic model is employed, an additional effect due to th114 becomes statistically significant and ynz90 and ju201 tend to become more so.

Table 3. t-Values for RFLP Markers on Chromosome 15 (Ns in parentheses)

Model	Marker								
	c15	cmw1	th114	dp151	ms114	efd49	ynz90	thh55	ju201
(1) Haseman—Elston									−1.86* (111)
(2) Augmented D-F			1.58 (40)				1.79* (54)		1.98* (111)
(3) D-F Basic: Selection (< 0)			−1.58 (12)				−1.19 (30)		−1.91* (44)
(4) D-F Basic: Selection (< −1)			−2.22* (11)				−2.82** (19)		−2.93*** (50)
(5) D-F Basic: Selection (< −2)			−2.26* (9)				−3.16*** (14)		−2.68*** (29)

* $p < 0.05$.
** $p < 0.01$.
*** $p < 0.005$.

The most noteworthy feature of the result of selection, however, is the marked tendency of the t-values to increase with selection. In these cases there is clearly a great increase in power with selection and this increase continues since, in spite of the decrease in sample size, the values of t either remain almost constant or increase. The analysis of the selected sample reaches high levels of significance for very modest sample sizes suggesting that the pessimism associated with the sib-pair method (Robertson, 1973) may be misplaced when selected samples are employed.

The fit of the basic model to data for marker ju201, which is the most informative marker available in this data set, is presented in more detail in Table 4. The expectation is that the basic model will detect an inverse linear relationship with the means of cosibs for probands of increasing values of $\hat{\pi}$. On the other hand probands' scores should show no relationship to $\hat{\pi}$. A fortuitous relationship is corrected for by the regression analysis. Table 4 shows precisely such a result with a degree of regularity unusual in real data. Probands show a reasonable uniformity of values but cosibs regress progressively back towards the population mean with smaller values of $\hat{\pi}$, with the single possible exception of $\hat{\pi}$ equal to 1.00, which is only based on a single sib pair. The table is instructive in illustrating the simple nature of the selected sample procedure. In essence it just involves a statistical comparison of the means in column five which have been corrected for discrepancies in the values $\overline{P}$ and with the average sib resemblance removed from the estimate of error.

Multivariate Analyses

A series of univariate analyses of the same phenotypic scores is less convincing than a multivariate one. Therefore, we repeated the analyses of

Table 4. Regression Selection Model (<0) Observed and Expected Co-sibling Means for Marker ju201

$$E(\overline{C}_s) = B_1\overline{P} + B_2\hat{\pi}_j + A$$

$$B_1 = -0.12 \quad B_2 = -1.75 \quad A = 0.31 \quad \overline{P} = -1.54$$

N	$\hat{\pi}$	$\overline{P}$	$\overline{C}$	$E(\overline{C}_s)$
1	0.00	−0.82	2.60	0.41
44	0.25	−1.21	−0.25	−0.02
35	0.50	−1.40	−0.94	−0.40
59	0.75	−1.20	−1.08	−0.86
1	1.00	−1.53	1.73	−1.26

Note: These Ns include the double entries required for the correct calculation of the means.

the selected samples entering the $\hat{\pi}$ simultaneously in a multiple regression equation. The results are shown in Table 5. Markers th114 and thh55 were excluded from this analysis because of insufficient sample sizes. The same two loci (ynz90 and ju201) manifest linkage with QTLs, but with somewhat increased significance.

DISCUSSION

It seems clear that the linkage analysis employing the DeFries and Fulker model is successful in terms of ease of application, substantial agreement with results of previous analyses, and a marked increase in power when used with selected samples. At least one QTL for reading disability is detected on chromosome 15, where we expected to find one, and with a very high level of significance even with quite small samples of selected probands. The method appears both reliable and powerful.

We have not presented systematic derivations of the models as these are discussed in detail in the literature cited. Neither have we presented systematic power calculations since the results are self evident in this respect. These calculations have been performed and it is hoped they will form the basis of a subsequent report (Carey and Williamson, in preparation) which considers other complications that we have ignored such as dominance and the effect of a single locus compared to that of several QTLs.

An approximate formula for calculating power for the analysis of selected samples and completely informative markers is

$$N = \frac{8(\text{non-central } \chi^2)(1 - R^2)}{[(\overline{P} - \mu)h^2]^2} \tag{7}$$

where $\overline{P}$ is the proband mean, μ is the population mean, h^2 is the heritability of the QTL, R is the overall sib correlation, and the non-central χ^2 is obtained from Pearson and Hartley (1972). N will be very sensitive to the degree of selection, $\overline{P} - \mu$, which is squared in the denominator of (7). Thus, small increases in selection have relatively large effects on power. The use of this formula gave the expected sample sizes shown in Table 6. These Ns seem roughly compatible with the levels of significance we obtained with the Ns in the present analyses.

In part, the effectiveness of these analyses could be due to the fact that the families from which the sibs pairs are drawn are few in number and selected for a high incidence of reading disability. The effect of such selection could lead to a few heterogeneous major locus systems, each segregating in only a few families or possibly only one family. In that case

Table 5. *t*-Values for RFLP Markers on Chromosome 15 for Multivariate Regression Selection Models (Ns in parentheses)

Model	Marker								
	c15	cmw1	th114	dp151	ms114	efd49	ynz90	thh55	ju201
(1) Multivariate Regression (<0)							−1.27 (20)		−1.18 (44)
(2) Multivariate Regression (<−1)							−4.41*** (19)		−4.68** (50)

Note: Markers th114 and thh55 omitted from analysis due to insufficient sample sizes.
** $p < 0.01$.
*** $p < 0.005$.

Table 6. Sib Pairs Needed to Reach Power of 0.50 and 0.90 for α levels 0.05 and 0.01 With Two Standard Deviations Selection Cutoff for Probands and Average Sib Correlations of 0.50

	$h^2 = 0.1$		$h^2 = 0.2$		$h^2 = 0.25$		$h^2 = 0.50$	
$1 - \beta$	0.50	0.90	0.50	0.90	0.50	0.90	0.50	0.90
α								
0.05	417	1148	104	287	51	137	16	46
0.01	717	1617	179	404	86	194	29	65

Note: For 3 SD cut off, divide Ns by 1.92.

the model would still provide a test for linkage, but the h^2 estimates would be higher than those typically found in the general population.

However, both our approximate power calculations and our substantive findings suggest that the regression approach applied to selected samples may have considerable utility in the detection of QTLs in behavioral and other human phenotypes.

ACKNOWLEDGEMENTS

This work was supported in part by program project and center grants from NICHD (HD-11681 and HD-27802) to J. C. DeFries.

NOTE

[1] Requests for the SAS files and accompanying documentation should be sent to Lon R. Cardon, Institute for Behavioral Genetics, University of Colorado, Boulder, Colorado 80309—0447, or by electronic mail to cardon@abacus.colorado.edu. No knowledge of SAS is required to run these programs.

REFERENCES

Blackwelder, W. C. and Elston, R. C. 1985. A comparison of sib-pair linkage tests for disease susceptibility loci. *Genetic Epidemiology, 2*, 85—97.

Cyphers, L. H., Phillips, K., Fulker, D. W., and Mrazek, D. A. 1990. Twin temperament during the transition from infancy to early childhood. *American Academy of Child and Adolescent Psychiatry, 29*, 392—397.

DeFries, J. C. 1985. Colorado reading project. In D. B. Gray and J. F. Kavanagh (eds.), *Biobehavioral Measures of Dyslexia* (pp. 123—135). Parkton, MD: York Press.

DeFries, J. C. and Fulker, D. W. 1985. Multiple regression analysis of twin data. *Behavior Genetics, 15*, 467—473.

DeFries, J. C. and Fulker, D. W. 1988. Multiple regression analysis of twin data: Etiology of deviant scores versus individual differences. *Acta Geneticae Medicae et Gemellologiae, 37,* 205—216.

DeFries, J. C., Olson, R. K., Pennington, B. F., and Smith, S. D. 1991. Colorado Reading Project: An update. In D. B. Gray and D. Duane (eds.), *The Reading Brain: The Biological Basis of Dyslexia.* Parkton, MD: York Press.

Dunn, L. M. and Markwardt, F. C. 1970. *Examiner's Manual: Peabody Individual Achievement Test.* Circle Pines, MN: American Guidance Service.

Haseman, J. K. and Elston, R. C. 1972. The investigation of linkage between a quantitative trait and a marker locus. *Behavior Genetics, 2,* 3—19.

Nance, W. E. and Neale, M. C. 1989. Partitioned twin analysis: A power study. *Behavior Genetics, 19,* 143—150.

Pearson, E. S. and Hartley, H. O. (eds.). 1972. *Biometrika Tables for Statisticians.* Cambridge: Cambridge University Press.

Robertson, A. 1973. Linkage between marker loci and those affecting a quantitative trait. *Behavior Genetics, 2,* 389—391.

SAS Institute, Inc. 1988. *SAS/STAT Users's Guide: Release 6.03 Edition.* Cary, NC: SAS Institute.

Smith, S. D., Kimberling, W. J., Pennington, B. F., and Lubs, H. A. 1983. Specific reading disability: Identification of an inherited form through linkage analysis. *Science, 219,* 1345—1347.

Cognitive and Academic Skills in Children with Sex Chromosome Abnormalities

BRUCE G. BENDER, MARY LINDEN and ARTHUR ROBINSON
National Jewish Center for Immunology and Respiratory Medicine, Denver, Colorado

ABSTRACT: Forty-six unselected children with various sex chromosome abnormalities (14 boys with 47,XXY, 4 boys with 47,XYY, 11 girls with 47,XXX, 9 girls with 45,X, and 8 girls with SCA mosaicism), identified through the consecutive chromosome screening of 40,000 Denver newborns, have been followed developmentally and evaluated in a protocol that included intellectual, language, and achievement testing. Controls consisted of 12 chromosomally normal males and 13 chromosomally normal females who were siblings of various propositi. While most SCA children were not mentally retarded, most of the nonmosaic propositi (31/37) received special education help for learning problems. In general, nonmosaic males were less severely affected than nonmosaic females, who demonstrated significantly reduced mean IQ scores on both Wechsler IQ tests. The inference that learning disorders were genetically mediated in this group was further supported by karyotype-specific findings. 47,XXY boys tended to demonstrate lower verbal skills and a specific reading disability. 47,XXX girls, while more globally impaired, demonstrated evidence of a specific weakness in language skills. 45,X girls tended to be globally impaired, but demonstrated a contrasting specific deficit in spatial thinking skills. Mosaic girls were not significantly different than controls on any measure, an outcome likely occurring because of the low percentage of aneuploid cells in these propositae. Variability was present in each group, and no single profile can characterize all children with any specific SCA. The presence of SCA, therefore, must be viewed as a risk factor creating a tendency towards LD but interacting with a host of other genetic and environmental forces to create a range of phenotypic outcomes.

KEYWORDS: children with sex chromosome abnormalities

Most research into the genetics of learning disabilities (LD) utilizes retrospective evaluation of LD children. This approach has utilized examination of familial patterns of transmission of reading disability (Smith, Kimberling, Pennington, and Lubs, 1983). Studies of monozygotic and dizygotic twins which include at least one reading disabled member provide even more accurate estimates of environmental and genetic contributions to the phenotype (DeFries, Fulker, and LaBuda, 1987). The possibility of identifying an LD subtype of specific genetic causation is significantly increased when a group of children with a known genetic abnormality can be identified and followed prospectively. The appearance of specific patterns of cognitive development, contrasted with control children also followed prospectively, allows more direct inference about the genetic origin of the resulting LD.

Reading and Writing: An Interdisciplinary Journal 3: 315—327, 1991.
© 1991 *Kluwer Academic Publishers.*

Approximately one in 200 newborns has a chromosome abnormality, and about half of these are sex chromosome abnormalities (SCA). SCAs are genetic anomalies involving an extra X or Y chromosome or a missing X chromosome and are associated with a variety of developmental disorders, but unlike more commonly seen autosomal abnormalities such as Down syndrome, children with SCA are more mildly affected. Learning disorders among SCA children are common (Bender, Puck, Salbenblatt, and Robinson, 1990; Pennington, Bender, Puck, Salbenblatt, and Robinson, 1982), although SCA likely accounts for less than 5% of LD children (Mutton and Lea, 1980; Friedrich, Dalby, Stachelin-Jensen, and Bruun-Peterson, 1982). The learning disorders of SCA children tend to be karyotype-specific; i.e., girls with an extra X chromosome have different cognitive abilities than boys with an extra X chromosome or girls who are missing an X chromosome (Bender, Linden, and Robinson, 1989; Linden, Bender, Harmon, Mrazek, and Robinson, 1988). The purpose of this report is to help define more clearly the LD phenotypes associated with SCAs.

METHOD

Subjects and Procedures

The Denver study of individuals with SCA was begun in 1964 by its principal investigator, Dr. Authur Robinson (Robinson and Puck, 1967). With the goal of determining the incidence of SCA in a newborn population, 40,000 consecutive newborns were screened for aneuploidy of the sex chromosomes by examining amniotic membranes of the placentas for Barr bodies. In the last 15,000 newborns, Wharton jelly from the transected umbilical cord was screened for Y bodies. Over 60 infants with various SCAs were thus identified and confirmed by chromosome analysis of peripheral blood cells.

Having thus identified this group of newborn propositi, it was decided to follow their development. The opportunity to study unselected individuals with SCA was particularly attractive given the confusion and controversy about these conditions. Earlier studies had determined that SCA individuals were over-represented in mental and penal institutions but provided little appreciation for the full spectrum of phenotypic expression. The Denver study, along with several other studies which began in various locations around the world, promised to provide a clearer picture of what happens to children born with SCA.

This prospective investigation has proceeded for the past 26 years, and the 46 propositi who have remained in the study are now in adolescence or early adulthood (Table 1). They include 14 boys with an extra X

Table 1. Denver study subjects

Karyotype	No. of subjects
47,XXY	14
47,XYY	4
47,XXX	11
45,X & VARIANTS	
45,X	6
46,XXq-	2
45,X/46,X,r(X)	1
FEMALE MOSAICS	
45,X/46,XX/47,XXX	1
45,X/46,XX	4
46,XX/47,XXX	1
45,X/47,XXX	2
46,XY CONTROLS	12
46,XX CONTROLS	13

chromosome, 4 boys with an extra Y chromosome, 11 girls with an extra X chromosome, 9 girls with X or partial X monosomy (referred to throughout this paper as the 45,X group), and 8 girls with SCA mosaicism. Our controls included 12 chromosomally normal males and 13 chromosomally normal females who are siblings of various propositi.

All children were seen at least once annually in our clinic for visits that included physical examinations and developmental and psychological testing. The battery of cognitive and academic measures are included in Table 2.

In addition to these laboratory-based measures, a history of special education intervention was collected through annual interviews with the children and their parents. In many cases, study personnel visited individual schools, meeting with school staff to discuss specific educational

Table 2. Cognitive and academic measures

Age	Test
4–5 years	Wechsler Preschool and Primary Scale of Intelligence
8–12 years	Wechsler Intelligence Scale for Children – Revised
	Composite Language Scale from Illinois Test of Psycholinguistic Ability
	Spatial Relations Test from Primary Mental Abilities Battery
	Peabody Individual Achievement Test: Reading Recognition Math

difficulties which had been encountered as well as to review planned interventions.

Results

Sample sizes for all karyotype groups are small. Because a normal distribution could not be established for some variables, paired comparisons between propositi and control groups were conducted with the Mann Whitney U Test ($p < 0.05$). All scores were converted to normative scale with mean of 100 and standard deviation of 15. In the case of the four 47,XYY boys, group data are included for inspection but we draw no conclusions.

Results for the Wechsler Preschool and Primary Scale of Intelligence (WPPSI), administered at four to five years of age, included a significantly reduced verbal IQ but not performance IQ in the 47,XXY group relative to the control group (Figure 1). The two groups of nonmosaic females, 47,XXX and 45,X, both had mean verbal and performance IQs lower than those of controls. However, the pattern in these two groups was notably different, with 45,X girls demonstrating relatively stronger verbal

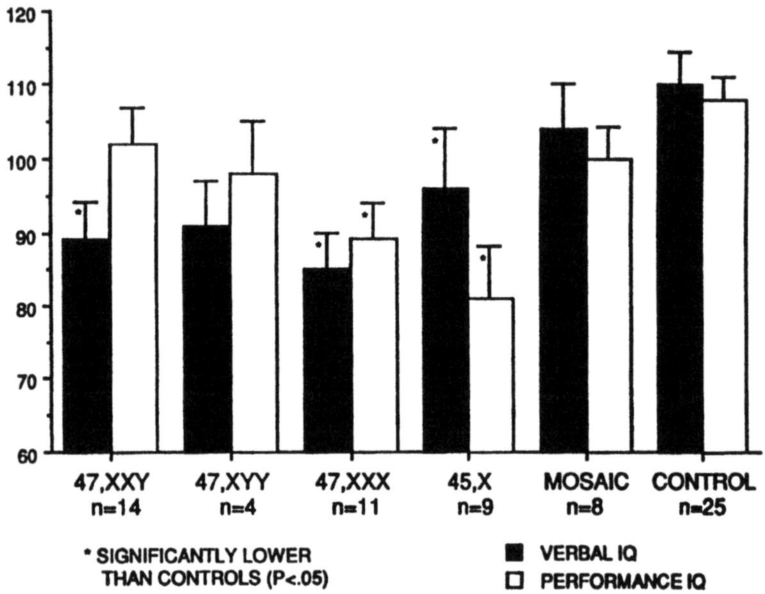

Fig. 1. Means and standard errors by group for the Wechsler Preschool and Primary Scale of Intelligence.

skills while the 47,XXX girls had depressed verbal as well as performance IQs. The mosaic girls did not differ from controls on either score.

Results from the Wechsler Intelligence Scale for Children — Revised (WISC-R), administered at eight years of age, included some similarities and some dissimilarities to the WPPSI results (Figure 2). In the 47,XXY group, the verbal and performance IQ means were essentially equal to each other and not significantly lower than controls. However, these results suggest mildly diminished general intellectual skills, and the absence of significant differences may be a matter of inadequate statistical power due to small sample size. As with the WPPSI scores, the WISC-R verbal and performance IQ means are significantly lower than controls for the two nonmosaic female groups. Just as the 47,XXY boys' verbal IQ < performance IQ discrepancy from the WPPSI gave way to fairly equal scores on the two halves of the WISC-R, so too the 45,X group's verbal IQ > performance IQ split on the WPPSI was absent in their WISC-R scores. Scores for the mosaic girls were again virtually identical to those of controls.

In addition to the intelligence test batteries, all subjects received two

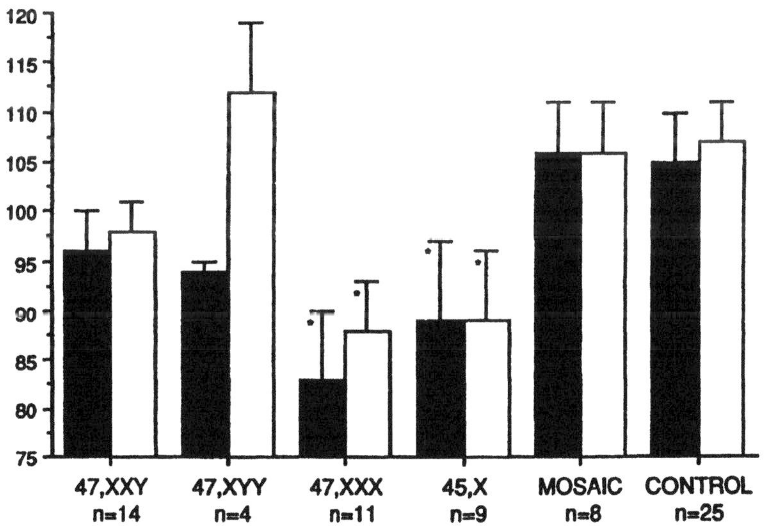

Fig. 2. Means and standard errors by group for the Wechsler Intelligence Scale for Children — Revised.

additional tests of cognitive abilities selected to compare and contrast language and spatial thinking skills across the karyotype groups (Figure 3). The 47,XXY boys did not differ significantly from controls on either of these tests (Figure 3). However, the pattern of results again suggests diminished language skills contrasted with relatively average spatial thinking skills. The 47,XXX group demonstrated depressed scores on both tests, although their greatest deficit appeared to emerge in language skills. The 45,X girls, in contrast, demonstrated significantly lower scores only on the test of spatial thinking. Scores of the mosaic group again did not differ from controls.

Mean scores from the reading recognition and math subtests of the Peabody Individual Achievement Test are seen in Figure 4. All three groups of nonmosaic propositi demonstrated significantly reduced reading scores. However, math scores were significantly reduced only in the 47,XXX and 45,X groups. Thus, while the nonmosaic females were uniformly deficient in math and reading, the 47,XXY boys were significantly deficient only in reading.

The incidence of specific LD requiring school intervention is represented in Table 3. The frequency rates are dramatically different for

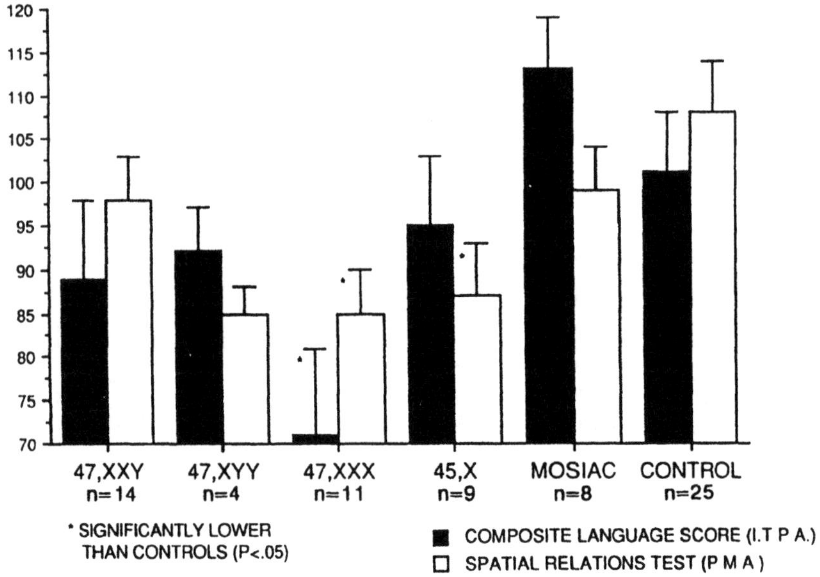

Fig. 3. Means and standard errors by group for the language and spatial relations tests.

Table 3. Incidence of specific learning disorders requiring educational intervention in propositi and controls as reported by elementary schools

	No Problem	Reading	Reading & Language	Math	Math & Language	All School Subjects	Mental Retardation
47,XXY ($N = 14$)	2	6	3			3	
47,XXY ($N = 4$)		2	2				
Male Controls ($N = 12$)	11	1					
47,XXX ($N = 11$)	2	1	3		3	1	1
45,X and Variants ($N = 9$)	3	1				4	1
Female Mosiacs ($N = 8$)	8						
Female Controls ($N = 13$)	11				1	11	

propositi and control children: 31 of 37 nonmosaic propositi received special education, in contrast to 4 of 25 controls. Among 47,XXY and 47,XYY boys, most educational assistance came in the form of part-time help for problems in reading and/or language difficulty, although three 47,XXY boys received placements in comprehensive intervention programs. The 47,XXX and 45,X groups received both limited reading/language as well as comprehensive intervention. However, half of these nonmosaic girls required broad, full-time intervention, and one from each group was diagnosed as mildly mentally retarded. No mosaic propositae received educational remediation.

DISCUSSION

While few SCA children are mentally retarded, the majority are LD. Hence, abnormalities of the sex chromosomes are a clearly identifiable, although not heritable, genetic etiology which can cause LD. Different abnormalities of the sex chromosomes can result in different patterns of cognitive development and different LDs. However, the cognitive phenotypes associated with the nonmosaic karyotypes — 47,XXY, 47,XYY, 47,XXX, and 45,X — are not discrete and markedly homogeneous. Variability is present in each group. For example, the standard deviations of mean IQ scores in each propositi group are very similar to standard deviations in the control group and the normative population. Consequently, IQ score ranges of 30 or more points are found in each SCA group. Scores on other cognitive tests include similar variability. The presence of SCA, therefore, must be viewed as a risk factor creating a tendency toward LD but interacting with a host of other genetic and environmental forces to create a range of phenotypic outcomes.

The finding of different cognitive development in different karyotype groups indicates that SCA does not produce a simple, singular effect such as reducing IQ by 50 points. Rather, different anomalies of the sex chromosomes tend to result in different types of LD, quite possibly because different sets of genes are altered. While these karyotype-specific LDs do not affect every child in every group, and not all studies report identical findings, cognitive profiles which characterize, to some degree, many SCA children within karyotype groups are now well established. The remaining discussion is directed at describing these cognitive phenotypes.

47,XXY. Approximately 1 in 600 newborn males has this karyotype. These boys, who as adults usually develop Klinefelter syndrome, frequently have impaired language skills, particularly in the area of expressive language (Bender et al., 1983). The cognitive test scores reported here also demonstrate weak composite language scores relative to fairly average spatial relations scores. In our group of 14 47,XXY boys, verbal IQ was lower than performance IQ in the preschool but not school age IQ results. However, pooled results from the international workshop (Netley, 1986)*, a group of six SCA investigations from four countries, indicated a strong general tendency for depressed verbal IQ. In the combined group of 73 47,XXY boys, mean Wechsler verbal IQ was 90 and performance IQ was 103 in contrast to control IQs of 102 and 104, respectively. In this pooled sample, 68% of propositi required educational intervention. While information about reading disability was not included for this international sample, two studies in addition to the Denver study evaluated reading. Ten of 15 47,XXY boys from Scotland required "reading remediation" (Ratcliffe, Murray, and Teague, 1986). Ten of 14 47,XXY boys in a Boston study "failed" a test of ability to read letter and word sounds, while other test results revealed significant deficits in phonic analysis which appeared to be responsible for their deficient reading and spelling skills (Graham, Bashir, Stark, Silbert, and Walzer, 1988). Results from both of

* The seven studies were from Denver, Colorado; Boston, Massachusetts; New Haven, Connecticut; Toronto and Winnipeg, Canada; Århus, Denmark; and Edinburgh, Scotland. Results reported here are included in the most recent publication from the international workshop (Ratcliffe and Paul, 1986), the third book in the series published by the March of Dimes Birth Defects Foundation.

these studies are consistent with the findings reported here and reveal reading disability in 47,XXY boys to be the most common, homogeneous LD found in any group of SCA children.

47,XYY. The inclusion of only four 47,XYY boys in our cohort occurred because the technology for identifying the smaller Y chromosome was not available until the final four years of newborn screening. Mild language delay was present in all four boys (Bender, Puck, Salbenblatt, and Robinson, 1984a), and all required part-time educational intervention for problems in reading or language and reading. A combined cohort of 28 47,XYY cases were reported by the international workshop (Netley, 1986). The incidence of 47,XYY is about on 1 in 1,000 newborn males. Mean verbal IQ (101) and performance IQ (109) were not significantly different from controls. Fifteen of 28 received educational intervention. Although the report from the international workshop did not include specific information about the type of educational intervention received, results from the largest single unselected cohort indicated that 8 of 16 47,XYY boys for whom school histories were available required "remedial teaching in reading" (Netley, 1986). Thus, the extra Y boys share with the extra X boys a marked tendency toward language and reading deficits and are frequently targeted by their schools for special education intervention. Along with these similarities, the two male groups also demonstrate differences. The average verbal IQ of the 47,XXY cohort appears to be about ten points lower than that of the 47,XYY cohort and, not surprisingly, they are selected for educational remediation somewhat more frequently. Therefore, while the 47,XYY karyotype may also be characterized to have an association with reading disability, this association seems less homogeneous than occurs among 47,XXY boys.

47,XXX. Girls with a 47,XXX karyotype, which occurs in about 1 in 1,200 female newborns, are as a group more intellectually impaired than any of the other three nonmosaic SCA groups. Their mean full scale IQ of 85 places them at the 15th percentile relative to the general population, and about 20 points lower than the control group. Nine of eleven triplo-X girls in our sample required special education; three of these were in full-time remedial classes, and a total of five required assistance in most school subjects. Although this group is below average in most cognitive skills, there is some evidence that they are most impaired in language abilities. Our test results included a composite language score considerably lower than the spatial relations test score, a pattern notably contrasting with the pattern shown in the 45,X group. The mean verbal IQ (87) of the cohort of 32 47,XXX girls from the international workshop was 8 points lower than their performance IQ (95), and 19 points lower than the control group verbal IQ. In that pooled cohort, 25 of the 35 propositae (71.4%)

for whom education histories were available received educational intervention (Netley, 1986).

45,X. The girls in this group do not have identical karyotypes, but each is missing part or all of an X chromosome and has physical stigmata consistent with Turner syndrome (Bender, Puck, Salbenblatt, and Robinson, 1984b). Both verbal and performance IQ were significantly reduced. More than half received school intervention in more than one subject, and three were in full-time special education classes. Although the 45,X group shares with the 47,XXX group a global impairment in cognitive abilities, the groups differ in two important ways. First, the 45,X group seems to be less generally deficient, as seen in the IQ and cognitive test scores, although their achievement test scores were similar. Second, the 45,X girls tend to demonstrate poorer spatial and performance scores but relatively better language scores. This visual/spatial deficit in Turner syndrome was first identified twenty-five years ago (Money and Alexander, 1966) and has been described extensively since (Bender et al., 1984b; Bender et al., 1990). Although the international workshop has not included a 45,X group, numerous investigators have reported associated deficits in orienting to left-right directions (Alexander, Walker, and Money, 1964), copying shapes (Silbert, Wolff, and Lilienthal, 1977), handwriting (Pennington et al., 1982), and solving math problems (Garron, 1977). Finally, our finding of broadly impaired cognitive ability is consistent with some reports of increased rates of mental retardation in Turner populations (Polani, 1960; Shaffer, 1962) but conflicts with more recent reports of reduced performance IQ but normal verbal IQ (McCauley, Kay, Ito, and Treder, 1987; Berch, Kirkendall, Briscoe, Digman, and Smith, 1985).

Mosaics. SCA mosaicism occurs where two or more cell lines with different karyotypes are found within a single individual. In our group of eight mosaic girls, half have 45,X/46,XX; that is, they have some cells with a normal (46,XX) and some with an abnormal (45,X) cell line. The remaining girls have some cells with a 47,XXX chromosome constitution. Generalizing about this genetically heterogeneous group is difficult. However, the proportion of abnormal cells in our group is less than 10%. Because this group does not differ from the controls on any cognitive or academic measure, it appears likely that their small proportion of aneuploid cells has not significantly affected their development. Reports from the international workshop included three different mosaic groups, two female and one male. No decreases in IQ or increases in educational intervention were found among the 11 45,X/46,XX mosaics, among the 5 46,XX/47,XXX mosaics, or among the 6 46,XY/47,XXY mosaics (Netley, 1986).

Other Abnormalities of the Sex Chromosomes

Although not included in the data reported here, other abnormalities of the sex chromosomes are known to occur. Individuals have been found to have three, four, and even five X chromosomes (49,XXXXX); men can have two Y chromosomes in combination with two X chromosomes (48,XXYY). In general, the addition of two or more extra sex chromosomes results in significantly increasing physical abnormality and intellectual impairment. Males with a 49,XXXXY chromosome constitution usually exhibit mental retardation and numerous physical stigmata, and may be mistaken for persons with Down syndrome (Nora and Fraser, 1981).

The fragile X syndrome also involves an abnormality of the sex chromosome but, unlike the other conditions described here, it does not result from the absence or addition of sex chromosomes. Fragile X is a common cause of X-linked mental retardation occurring in approximately 1 in 1,000 male births and recognized by a marker, or fragile site, consisting of a constriction on the long arm of the X chromosome. This

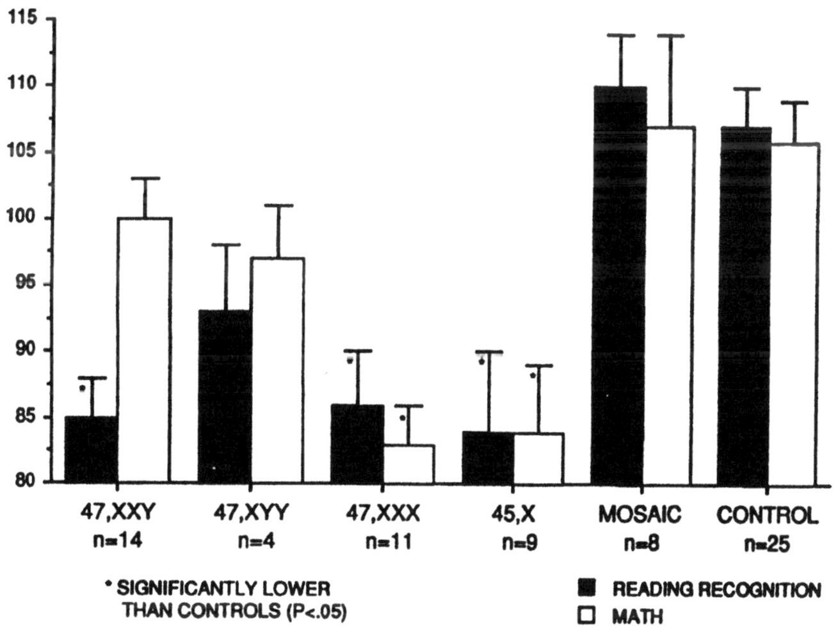

Fig. 4. Means and standard errors by group for the reading recognition and math subtests from the Peabody Individual Achievement Test.

abnormality is thus a combination of a mutant gene or genes associated with a specific cytogenetic anomaly. Only males have fragile X syndrome because they have only one X chromosome, while females, with two X chromosomes, are partially protected if one of their X chromosomes carries the marker. However, some fragile X positive female do demonstrate cognitive and behavioral impairments which apparently result from their genetic defect (Hagerman and McBogg, 1983). While these girls are not as likely to be mentally retarded as the fragile X males, they have lower IQs and increased incidence of learning disorders. The fragile X positive females, then, may be quite similar to the two groups of nonmosaic SCA females, those missing an X and those with an extra X. Together, these three groups of females are likely to increase our understanding of the role of the X chromosome and the genes it carries in normal and abnormal cognitive development, and will further elucidate how genetic etiologies can create LDs in some children.

REFERENCES

Alexander, D., Walker, H. T., and Money, J. 1964. Studies in direction sense: I. Turner's syndrome. *Archives of General Psychiatry, 10*, 337–339.

Bender, B., Fry, E., Pennington, B., Puck, M., Salbenblatt, J., and Robinson, A. 1983. Speech and language development in 41 children with sex chromosome anomalies. *Pediatrics, 71*, 262–267.

Bender, B., Puck, M., Salbenblatt, J., and Robinson, A. 1984a. Cognitive development of unselected girls with complete and partial X monosomy. *Pediatrics, 73*, 175–182.

Bender, B., Puck, M., Salbenblatt, J., and Robinson, A. 1984b. The development of four unselected 47,XYY boys. *Clin. Genet., 25*, 435–445.

Bender, B., Linden, M., and Robinson, A. 1989. Verbal and spatial processing efficiency in 32 children with sex chromosome abnormalities. *Pediatric Research, 25*, 577–579.

Bender, B., Puck, M., Salbenblatt, J., and Robinson, A. 1990. Cognitive development of children with sex chromosome abnormalities. *In* C. S. Holmes (ed.), *Psychoneuroendocrinology: Brain, Behavior, and Hormonal Interactions* (pp. 138–163). New York: Springer-Verlag.

Berch, D. B., Kirkendall, K. L., Briscoe, G., Digman, P. S. J., and Smith, K. L. 1985. Spatial information processing in children with Turner's syndrome. *Presented at the Society for Research in Child Development Meeting, Toronto.*

DeFries, J. C., Fulker, D. W., and LaBuda, M. C. 1987. Evidence for a genetic aetiology in reading disability of twins. *Nature, 329*, 537–539.

Friedrich, V., Dalby, M., Stachelin-Jensen, T., and Bruun-Peterson, G. 1982. Chromosome studies of children with developmental language retardation. *Developmental Medicine Child Neurology, 24*, 645–652.

Garron, D. C. 1977. Intelligence among persons with Turner's syndrome. *Behavioral Genetics, 7*, 105–127.

Graham, J. M., Bashir, A. S., Stark, R. E., Silbert, A., and Walzer, S. 1988. Oral and written language abilities of XXY boys: Implications for anticipatory guidance. *Pediatrics, 81*, 795–806.

Hagerman, R. J. and McBogg, P. M. 1983. The Fragile X Syndrome: Diagnosis, Biochemistry, and Intervention. Dillon, CO: Spectra Publishing.

Linden, M., Bender, B., Harmon, R., Mrazek, D., and Robinson, A. 1988. 47,XXX: What is the prognosis? *Pediatrics, 82,* 619—630.
McCauley, E., Kay, T., Ito, J., and Treder, R. 1987. The Turner syndrome: Cognitive deficits, affective discrimination, and behavior problems. *Child Development, 58,* 464—473.
Money, J. and Alexander, D. 1966. Turner syndrome: Further demonstration of the presence of specific congential deficiencies. *Journal of Medical Genetics, 3,* 47—48.
Mutton, D. E. and Lea, J. 1980. Chromosome studies of children with specific speech and language delay. *Developmental medicine and child neurology, 22,* 588—594.
Netley, C. 1986. Summary overview of behavioral development in individuals with neonatally identified X and Y aneuploidy. *Birth Defects: Original Article Series, 22,* 293—306.
Nora, J. J. and Fraser, F. C. 1981. *Medical Genetics: Principles and Practice.* Philadelphia: Lea and Febiger.
Pennington, B. F., Bender, B., Puck, M., Salbenblatt, J., and Robinson, A. 1982. Learning disabilities in children with sex chromosome anomalies. *Child Development, 53,* 1182—1192.
Polani, P. E. 1960. Chromosomal factors in certain types of educational subnormality. *In* P. W. Bowman and H. B. Mautner (eds.), *Mental Retardation: Proceedings of the First International Congress* (pp. 421—438). New York: Grune and Stratton.
Ratcliffe, S. G., Murray, L., and Teague, P. 1986. Edinburgh study of growth and development of children with sex chromosome abnormalities. III. *Birth Defects: Original Article Series, 22,* 73—118.
Ratcliffe, S. and Paul, N. (eds.). 1986. Prospective Studies on Children With Sex Chromosome Aneuploidy. *Birth Defects: Original Article Series, 22.* New York: Alan R. Liss.
Robinson, A. and Puck, T. 1967. Studies on chromosomal nondisjunction in man, II. *American Journal of Human Genetics, 19,* 112—129.
Shaffer, J. W. 1962 A specific cognitive deficit observed in gonadal aplasia (Turner's syndrome). *Journal of Clinical Psychology, 18,* 403—406.
Silbert, A., Wolff, P. H., and Lilienthal, J. 1977. Spatial and temporal processing in patients with Turner's syndrome. *Behavioral Genetics, 7,* 11—21.
Smith, S. D., Kimberling, W. J., Pennington, B. F., and Lubs, H. A. 1983. Specific reading disability: Identification of an inherited form through linkage analysis. *Science, 219,* 1345—1347.

Neurology/Neuropsychology

Planum Temporale Asymmetry: In-Vivo Morphometry Affords a New Perspective for Neuro-Behavioral Research

HELMUTH STEINMETZ [1] and ALBERT M. GALABURDA [2]

[1] *Department of Neurology, Heinrich-Heine-University, Moorenstr. 5, D-4000 Düsseldorf 1, Germany;* [2] *Department of Neurology, Harvard Medical School, Boston, MA, and Neurological Unit and Charles A. Dana Research Institute, Beth Israel Hospital, 330 Brookline Avenue, Boston, MA 02215, U.S.A.*

ABSTRACT: High-resolution magnetic resonance (MR) imaging today allows the *in vivo* quantification of the surface area of the cortex covering the planum temporale and permits assessment of the direction and degree of individual left-right asymmetry of this structure. This methodologic advance is promoting new studies on the biological mechanisms of anatomic and functional lateralization and on the structural accompaniments of disorders such as developmental dyslexia. It is important to stress that studies must agree on the definition and measurement of planum asymmetry, and we review our definition and its justification in the present article.

Data obtained from normal subjects supported the assumption that planum (a)symmetry underlies functional lateralization. Thus, familial sinistrality predicted for symmetry of the planum in all eight left-handers studied. The pattern of planum symmetry in the normals was similar to that found in the *post mortem* studies of dyslexic individuals. Insofar as hand preference and developmental dyslexia are in part genetically transmitted, we suggest that planum symmetry may represent an inherited condition as well. Furthermore, even though planum symmetry is part of the anatomic substrate of developmental dyslexia, it is unlikely that it represents a form of developmental anatomic pathology.

KEYWORDS: Dyslexia; Reading; Handedness; Laterality; Temporal lobe; Planum temporale; Magnetic resonance imaging.

INTRODUCTION

Until recently, convincing evidence that left-right asymmetry of the planum temporale underlies functional lateralization (Geschwind and Levitsky 1968; Galaburda *et. al.* 1978a, 1987; Geschwind and Galaburda 1987) was not obtainable because planum morphometry was only possible *post mortem* when functional measures were seldom available. However, the following findings suggested a structural-functional relationship: (1) On the left side, the planum lies at the center of "Wernicke's speech area" (Geschwind 1970), for which left hemisphere dominance has been established in the majority of individuals; (2) the planum is covered mostly by auditory association cortex, which is thought to play a role in language processing (von Economo and Horn 1930; Galaburda *et al.* 1978a, b;

Reading and Writing: An Interdisciplinary Journal **3**: 331—343, 1991.
© 1991 *Kluwer Academic Publishers.*

Galaburda and Sanides 1980) (fig. 1); (3) phylogenetically, the planum temporale is clearly visible first in the human brain, which suggests a relationship to the evolution of language (Yeni-Komshian and Benson 1976); (4) fourteen postmortem studies consistently demonstrated the left planum area to be larger than the right in the majority of adult, fetal and neonatal brains (Steinmetz *et al.* 1990b); (5) asymmetry of the planum correlated with cytoarchitectonic asymmetries of auditory association area Tpt (Galaburda *et al.* 1978b) and parietal area PG (Eidelberg and Galaburda 1984), both of which are areas that can be involved by lesions that lead to aphasic disorders; and (6) positron emission tomography demonstrated a left-lateralized increase in glucose metabolism or cerebral blood flow in the region of Heschl's gyrus and the planum temporale upon verbal auditory stimulation (Mazziotta *et al.* 1982; Petersen *et al.* 1988).

Several methods have been employed for showing the planum temporale in *post mortem* specimens, which are not the focus of this discussion and will not be outlined in detail. The original assessment by Geschwind and Levitsky (1968) was made from dissected temporal lobes that had been photographed from above and the outer lengths of the plana measured linearly. One of us (AMG) has published on autopsy specimens that had been embedded and serially sectioned for histologic analysis. It was necessary in this serially sectioned material to reconstruct the plana before measurements could be made. This was accomplished either optically with the use of a distortion-free projection apparatus, or by means of a computer program that reconstructed the plana from digitized images of the sections. After reconstructions, the surface area of the plana was measured by perimetry or with the computer system. In these cases all portions of the posterior Sylvian fossa were taken into consideration, from H2 rostrally (see below and figure 2) until the caudal end, to include the terminal limb of the ascending ramus.

Absence of planum asymmetry was a consistent finding in the brains of six male and three female dyslexic individuals consecutively studied at autopsy (Galaburda and Kemper 1979; Galaburda *et al.* 1985; Humphreys *et al.* 1990). Generally, absence of planum asymmetry reflects an excessive development of the ordinarily smaller planum, thus providing two relatively large plana as opposed to only one relatively large planum in the asymmetric case (Galaburda *et al.* 1987). In animal models, symmetric architectonic areas as compared to asymmetric homologous area, contain an excess of neurons (Galaburda *et al.* 1986), as well as an expansion of the region containing interhemispheric connections (Rosen *et al.* 1989). The functional significance of these anatomic consequences of symmetry has not been studied, but it remains likely that such changes in cellular and connectional architecture are accompanied by differences in functional capacity.

Minor cortical malformations (microgyria and/or microdysgenesis) or other manifestations of early cortical injury have also been reported in the same autopsy studies (Galaburda and Kemper 1979; Galaburda *et al.* 1985; Humphreys *et al.* 1990). However, some of these abnormalities have also been seen in non-dyslexics (Kaufmann and Galaburda 1989; Humphreys *et al.* 1990). Similar abnormalities in experimental animals (for instance, see Sherman *et al.* 1985, 1990 a, b, and c; Humphreys *et al.* 1991; Innocenti and Berbel in press a and b) are associated with substantial reorganization of the cortex, including abnormal numbers of some types of neurons and abnormal afferent and efferent connections.

Since planum symmetry is present in 25% of randomly selected individuals (containing both dyslexics and nondyslexics), this factor could not alone explain the presence of dyslexia. One possibility to consider is that anatomic symmetry is a non-pathologic condition that prevents functional compensation for the cortical pathology seen in dyslexic patients. A related alternative is that planum symmetry, though non-pathological, imposes a limit on the number and types of linguistic strategies (see, Bever *et al.* 1989), which in turn are further inhibited by the presence of developmental cortical lesions. Symmetry alone or developmental cortical anomalies alone would by these hypotheses not be expected to result in functional changes. In both hypotheses planum symmetry is seen as manifestation of normal variation and only the cortical dysgenesis represents true developmental pathology. Moreover, there may be independent genetic influences for both types of anatomic findings, the normal and abnormal one, since we have found them to occur separately in *post mortem* brains (Kaufmann and Galaburda 1989; Humphreys *et al.* 1990).

Still another explanation would imply that anatomic symmetry can be the pathologic consequence of lesion-induced abnormal corticogenesis (c.f., Goldman-Rakic and Rakic 1984). In other words, early cortical injury that leads to cortical dysgenesis produces secondary reorganization of the planum in favor of greater symmetry. Or, it may be that both planum symmetry and developmental cortical lesions are pathologic consequences of a third factor or factors, but that they are not causally related. In either of these two circumstances the two separate pathologic findings coincide in the same individual in order for dyslexic symptoms to appear. However, if either of these situations were to be correct, and the planum symmetry represents true pathology, then it could require large samples to demonstrate familial influences on individual planum temporale (a)symmetry since multiple causes, some of which are not familial, could conceivably lead to the initial cortical insult.

In this paper, we will discuss recent magnetic resonance (MR) imaging findings in healthy individuals relating planum symmetry to anomalous

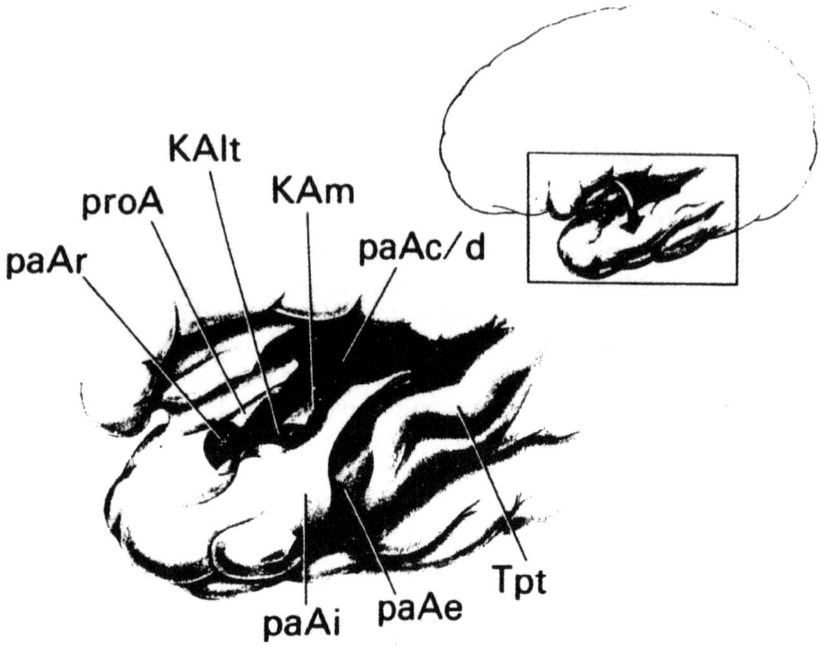

Fig. 1: Semistylized diagram of the superior temporal region of the human brain, covered by the auditory representation (from Galaburda 1984). Cytoarchitectonic areas KAm und KAlt represent the primary auditory koniocortex, mainly located on the anterior transverse gyrus of Heschl. Areas designated "pa" are the parakoniocortical (association cortex) belts (Galaburda and Sanides 1980). Slightly more homotypical auditory association area Tpt covers the posterolateral aspect of the planum temporale and posterior superior temporal gyrus and shows an individually variable "spill" onto the lateral aspect of the parietal opercular cortex. Nevertheless, left-right asymmetry of area Tpt parallels gross asymmetry of the planum (Galaburda *et al.* 1978b).

functional lateralization, which shows a strong familial influence. We will also describe our morphometric protocol, which we hope will be widely implemented in future studies.

ANATOMIC DEFINITION OF THE PLANUM TEMPORALE

A variety of definitions of the anterior and posterior anatomic borders of the planum has been used by previous investigators. According to cytoarchitectonic and myelogenetic data (von Economo and Horn 1930; Galaburda and Sanides 1980; Pfeifer 1936), we define the *anterior border* of the planum as Heschl's sulcus, i.e., the transverse sulcus bordering the anterior transverse temporal gyrus posteriorly (the anterior transverse temporal gyrus is identified by "Pfeifer's criterion", i.e., by a prominent medial origin immediately behind the insula; see fig. 2). This definition of the anterior border of the planum is reliable between observers (Steinmetz *et al.* 1989b).

The controversy regarding the *posterior border* of the planum has entailed the question of whether or not to include the posterior wall of the terminal ascending ramus of the Sylvian fissure (which belongs to the supramarginal gyrus). It is fair to state that the limit between the rostral and terminal portions of this segment of the Sylvian fissure is not sharp.

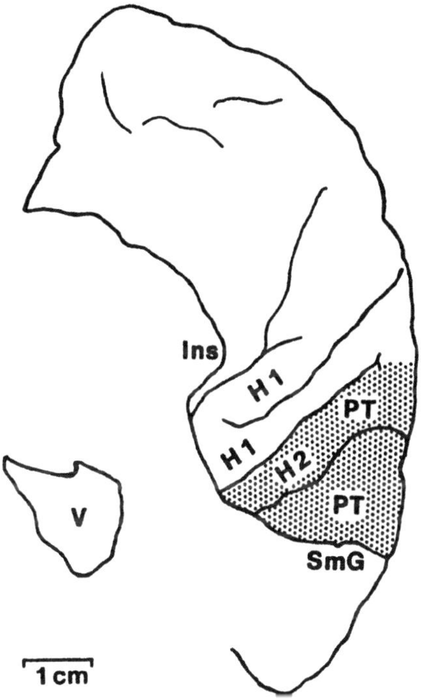

Fig. 2.: Anatomic definition of the anterior border of the planum temporale; diagram is of the aerial view of the upper surface of a dissected right temporal lobe (from Steinmetz *et al.* 1990b): H1 — anterior or first transverse gyrus of Heschl; H2 — second transverse gyrus of Heschl; PT — planum temporale (shaded area, which includes H2); SmG — supramarginal gyrus; Ins — insula; V — ventricle. In this illustrative case, four "transverse" sulci are seen on the supratemporal plane. Of them, three commence from the medial retroinsular space and are transverse sulci proper (Pfeifer's criterion). However, only the first and second transverse sulcus border H1 anteriorly and posteriorly respectively. The second transverse sulcus is also called "Heschl's sulcus", i.e., the anterior border of the planum. The third transverse sulcus borders H2 posteriorly and is part of the planum. Note that H1 is split by an intermediate sulcus which is *not* a transverse sulcus according to Pfeifer's criterion. A clear understanding of supratemporal sulcus patterns is crucial for reliable planum measurements.

Von Economo and Horn (1930) excluded terminal portion form their planum measurements, whereas Geschwind and Levitsky (1968) included it in theirs (fig. 3). Measurements using the Geschwind and Levitsky definition tend to lessen the degree of left-right asymmetry, since the ascending ramus is usually more pronounced on the right side (Rubens *et al.* 1976; Steinmetz *et al.* 1990b). In the architectonic study of Galaburda and Sanides (1980) auditory association are Tpt continues posteriorly to the end of the Sylvian fissure on both sides, thus not distinguishing between the rostral and terminal portions, and sometimes goes beyond onto the parietal operculum on the left (Galaburda, Sanides and Geschwind, 1978b; see figure 1). This would suggest that the terminal portion

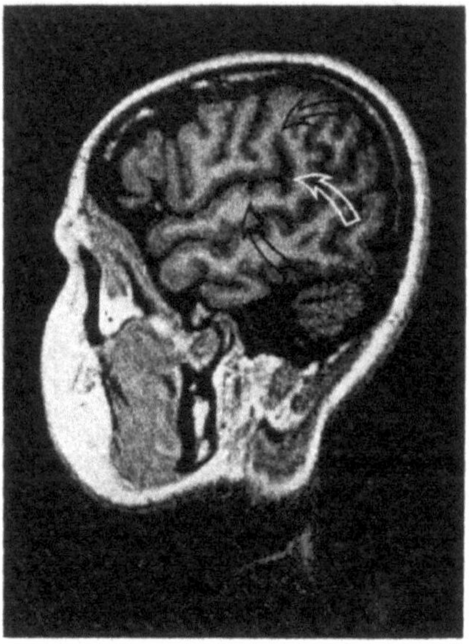

Fig. 3: In-vivo MR morphometry of the planum temporale (FLASH-MR sequence); the figure displays one slice out of a total of 128 contiguous sections obtained from each brain. Thickness of each slice is 1.17 mm with a sagittal imaging plane, avoiding partial volume effects. Planum morphometry then measures the curved length of the planum on all slices, thereby controling for individual variability of cortical folding (Steinmetz *et al.* 1990b and 1991). The figure shows a sagittal cut through a right hemisphere with a small planum; anterior is on the left of the figure. The *left arrow* marks the bottom of Heschl's sulcus, i.e., the anterior border of the planum. The gyral elevations left and right of Heschl's sulcus on the supratemporal plane are the first (H1) and second (H2) transverse gyri, respectively (compare with figures 1 and 2). The *right lower (white) arrow* marks the end of the horizontal segment of the Sylvian fissure, i.e., the posterior border of the planum with the von Economo and Horn (1930) definition (See text). The *right upper* arrow marks the end of the terminal ascending ramus of the Sylvian fissure, i.e., the posterior border of the planum within the Geschwind and Levitsky (1968) definition. See text for technical MR data.

should be included in measurements of the planum. However (*see below*), functional data may favor the von Economo and Horn definition.

Definition of the *lateral* and *medial borders* of the planum has been uniform among previous investigators. The lateral border is the superolateral rim of the superior temporal gyrus, and the medial border is the retroinsular point where the anterior and posterior limits of the planum coincide (fig. 2).

IN-VIVO MR MORPHOMETRY

High-resolution volume imaging of the brain has recently become available with the gradient echo MR sequences. The fast low-angle shot ("FLASH") sequence generates contiguous brain slices as thin as 1 mm, with excellent gray matter-white matter contrast (fig. 3), and without important image distortion (Filipek *et al.* 1989; Steinmetz *et al.* 1989b, 1990b; for additional technical information, *see below*). Using image processing software, FLASH-datasets allow volume measurements of the whole brain (Filipek *et al.* 1989), or surface area measurements of individual brain regions, such as the planum temporale (Steinmetz *et al.* 1990b, 1991). For the first time in human brain science, MR morphometry provides direct correlations between relatively fine-grained structural observations and behavioral or genetic data. It also avoids some problems of *post mortem* studies, such as fixation artifacts or long intervals between functional and morphologic examinations.

Prior to image acquisition, the patient's head is fixed with foam rubber in the MR head coil to avoid movement. According to axial and coronal fast locating scans, the head is then repositioned and re-fixed until the midsagittal plane of the brain is aligned in parallel with the sagittal imaging plane (Steinmetz *et al.* 1989a, 1990a). Technical data of the volumetric FLASH sequence, which follows thereafter, are 40 msec repetition time, 5 msec echo time, 40 degrees flip angle, 1 excitation, 25 cm field of view, 256 × 256 image matrix, 15 cm thickness of the excited volume, 128 partitions, and 22 minutes measuring time (1.5 Tesla Magnetom/circulary polarized head coil manufactured by Siemens, D-8520 Erlangen, Germany). This sequence provides 128 contiguous sagittal slices of 1.17 mm single slice thickness and 1 × 1 mm pixel size (fig. 3). Morphometry of the planum is performed off-line using simple software of our own design that allows curved length measurements and has been implemented on a commercial image processing workstation (Steinmetz *et al.* 1990b). Progressing image by image from medial to lateral slices, a cursor is manually traced within the gray matter of the planum, following all gyral and sulcal outlines from the anterior until the posterior border (fig. 3). Length measurements on single slices are automatically summed with those from the previous sections and multiplied by the slice thickness. Thereby, morphometry measures the *total* surface area and controls for individual variability of cortical folding (Steinmetz *et al.* 1990b). Anatomic left-right asymmetry is expressed as the asymmetry coefficient (R−L)/[0.5(R+L)], where R and L are the planum areas on the right and left hemispheres, respectively. The coefficient corrects for variability in brain size (Eidelberg and Galaburda, 1984; Galaburda *et al.* 1987). Negative values indicate leftward asymmetry; positive values rightward asymmetry. Planum measurements referred to in this article were performed by one "blinded" observer (HS). High interobserver reliability using the above anatomic criteria has been demonstrated in previous methodologic studies (Steinmetz *et al.* 1989b).

FACTORS INFLUENCING PLANUM ASYMMETRY IN HEALTHY SUBJECTS

MR morphometry has recently provided the first empirical support for the hypotheses that planum (a)symmetry is an anatomic substrate of functional lateralization (Geschwind and Levitsky 1968; Galaburda *et al.* 1978a), and that anatomic asymmetry is modulated by prenatal factors that also co-modulate hemispheric dominance (Geschwind and Galaburda 1987). Thus, in a MR study, Steinmetz and coworkers (1991) showed that left-handers (LH) have a lesser degree of leftward planum asymmetry than right-handers (RH). Among twenty LH, eight who had sinistral first-degree relatives comprised a subgroup with symmetric plana (figs. 4 and 5). Although language lateralization was unknown in these healthy subjects, the data suggest that planum symmetry is a substrate of atypical language dominance, since right hemisphere or bilateral representation of language is especially frequent in LH with familial sinistrality (Hécaen *et al.* 1981).

It is worth noting that the anatomic difference between LH and RH was significant only when the von Economo and Horn definition of the planum temporale was used. Extension of planum measurements to include the posterior wall of the terminal ascending Sylvian ramus (the Geschwind and Levitsky definition) reduced overall degree of left-right asymmetry, and failed to detect significant group differences. Thus, functional asymmetries may be more closely related to the asymmetric angulation of the Sylvian fissures on the two sides than to an asymmetry of the total amount of posterior intrasylvian cortex. Conversely, the exclusion of the terminal segment may artificially enhance an asymmetry that is already present with the segment included, and this enhancement may permit the detection of differences in relatively small groups. In other words, with larger samples, it would be possible that the inclusion of the terminal portion would still lead to statistically significant differences between LH

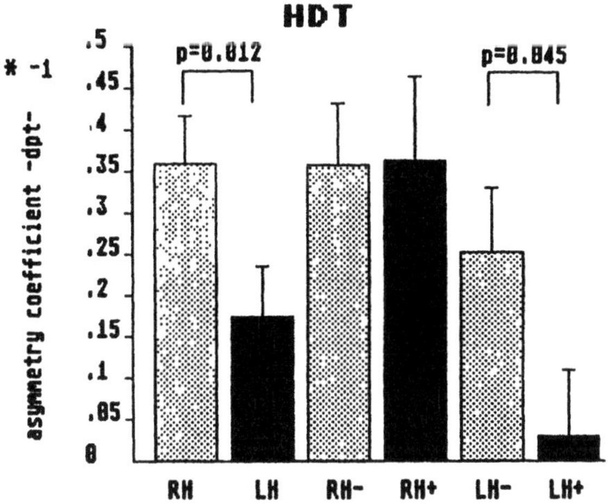

Fig. 4: Means and standard errors of the degrees of leftward planum asymmetry in 29 right-handers (RH) and 20 left-handers (LH) with (RH+, LH+) or without (RH–, LH–) familial sinistrality among first-degree relatives; y-axis: anatomic asymmetry coefficient $[(R - L)/ 0.5 (R + L)] * -1$ indicating degree of leftward asymmetry; HDT: hand-dominance-test of motor proficiency, which was used as handedness criterion (Steingrüber 1971). Two-sided p-values < 0.05 were significant (Mann-Whitney U-test). Note that leftward planum asymmetry is reduced in LH compared to RH, and in LH+ compared to LH– (Steinmetz 1991).

and RH groups. These results establish a correlation between familial sinistrality and the finding of individual symmetry of the planum temporale. It is likely, therefore, that a normal hereditary factor plays a role in the anatomic expression of symmetry of the planum.

FUTURE RESEARCH

As illustrated by figures 4 and 5, qualitative statements such as "left larger" or "right larger" would miss a crucial point in future investigations on structural-functional relationships in cerebral (a)symmetry. Structural asymmetries are distributed along a continuum of individual degrees (as are functional asymmetries). Rather than the category, it is the degree of "left larger" which will make an anatomic difference between functionally, genetically, or sex defined populations. Twin and family studies are needed to investigate the question of heritability of planum (a)symmetry. It remains likely that magnitude of planum asymmetry, whether symmetric, slightly asymmetric, or strongly asymmetric, will be shown to be heritable. This is in contrast to directionality of asymmetry, e.g., left larger versus right larger. There is a body of evidence in the experimental literature that

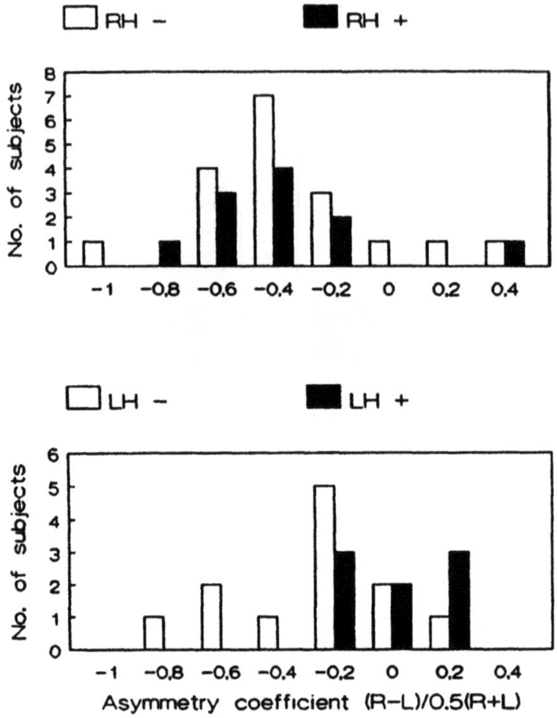

Fig. 5: Distribution of individual degrees of planum asymmetry in the same subjects as figure 4. Negative values on the x-axis indicate leftward planum asymmetry; positive values, rightward asymmetry. Note that LH with familial sinistrality (LH+) form a homogenous, anatomically symmetric subgroup (Steinmetz 1991).

supports this hypothesis. Thus, for example, Collins (1981) has shown that it is possible to breed rats for strength of pawedness but not for direction. In as far as we can tell at present, the only difference between dyslexic and nondyslexic brains, *vis-à-vis* planum (a)symmetry, is that the former show lack of asymmetry rather than reversal in directionality. In that case, it becomes more likely that symmetry in dyslexic as well as in the general population reflects a heritable factor.

In the past, neuroradiologic studies of dyslexic patients have used relatively crude or arbitrary measures of structural asymmetry, such as anterior or posterior hemisphere widths (Hier *et al.* 1978; Haslam *et al.* 1981; Hynd *et al.* 1990), temporal lobe volumes (Rumsey *et al.* 1986), or planum lengths assessed on extreme lateral sagittal MR sections (Hynd *et al.* 1990). However, hemisphere widths, for example, have been of questionable functional significance in non-dyslexic populations (Henderson *et al.* 1984). Investigations of well-defined cortical regions with known functional contributions, e.g., the planum and the corpus callosum, appear more promising for elucidating structural-functional relationships in normal and abnormal brains. The proposed MR protocol will allow for evaluations of effects of zygosity on planum (a)symmetry, the effect of gender, the effect of age, particularly related to the question of degenerative disorders associated with language deficits (Mesulam 1982), and the effect of known chromosomal aberrations and identified gene loci on the expression of planum size and (a)symmetry. Prior to failure in schools useful associations between planum morphology and (a)symmetry might be used as markers of risk for the development of language disorders in children from families in which these disorders are present.

ACKNOWLEDGEMENT

The work reported here was supported in part by grants from the Deutsche Forschungsgemeinschaft (SFB 200/Z2 and 194/A7) to HS and by NIH grants (HD 20806, 19819 and NS 27119-01A2), grant from the Carl W. Herzog Foundation, and a grant from the Research Division of the Orton Dyslexia Society to AMG.

REFERENCES

Bever, T. G., Carrithers, C., Cowart, W. and Townsend, D. J. (1989). Language processing and familial handedness. In A. M. Galaburda (ed.), *From Reading to Neurons.* Cambridge: Bradford Books/MIT Press, 331—360.

Collins, R. L. (1981). A demonstration of an inheritance of the direction of asymmetry that is consistent with the notion that genetic alleles are left-right indifferent. *Behavioral Genetics, 11,* 596—600.

von Economo, C. and Horn, L. (1930). Über Windungsrelief, Masse und Rindenarchitektonik der Supratemporalfläche, ihre individuellen und ihre Seitenunterschiede. *Zeitschrift für Neurologie und Psychiatrie, 130,* 678—757.

Eidelberg, D. and Galaburda, A. M. (1984). Inferior parietal lobule. Divergent architectonic asymmetries in the human brain. *Archives of Neurology, 41,* 843—852.

Filipek, P. A., Kennedy, D. N., Caviness, V. S., Rossnick, S. L., Spraggins, T. A. and Starewicz, P. M. (1989). Magnetic resonance imaging-based brain morphometry: development and application to normal subjects. *Annals of Neurology, 25,* 61—67.

Galaburda, A. M., LeMay, M., Kemper, T. and Geschwind, N (1978a). Right-left asymmetries in the brain. Structural differences between the hemispheres may underlie cerebral dominance. *Science, 199,* 852—856.

Galaburda, A. M., Sanides, F. and Geschwind, N. (1978b). Human brain. Cytoarchitectonic left-right asymmetries in the temporal speech region. *Archives of Neurology, 35,* 812—817.

Galaburda, A. M. and Kemper, T. L. (1979). Cytoarchitectonic abnormalities in developmental dyslexia: a case study. *Annals of Neurology, 6,* 94—100.

Galaburda, A. M. and Sanides, F. (1980). Cytoarchitectonic organization of the human auditory cortex. *Journal of Comparative Neurology, 190*, 597—610.

Galaburda, A. M. (1984). Anatomical asymmetries. In N. Geschwind and A. M. Galaburda (eds.), *Cerebral dominance. The Biological Foundations*. Cambridge: Harvard University Press, 11—25.

Galaburda, A. M., Sherman, G. F., Rosen, G. D., Aboitiz, F. and Geschwind N. (1985). Developmental dyslexia: four consecutive patients with cortical anomalies. *Annals of Neurology, 18*, 222—233.

Galaburda, A. M., Aboitiz, F., Rosen, G. D. and Sherman, G. F. (1986). Historical asymmetry in the primary visual cortex of the rat: implications for mechanisms of cerebral asymmetry. *Cortex, 22*, 151—160.

Galaburda, A. M., Corsiglia, J., Rosen, G. D. and Sherman, G. F. (1987). Planum temporale asymmetry, reappraisal since Geschwind and Levitsky. *Neuropsychologia, 25*, 853—868.

Geschwind, N. and Levitsky, W. (1968). Human brain: Left-right asymmetries in temporal speech region. *Science, 161*, 186—187.

Geschwind, N. (1970). The organization of language and the brain. *Science, 170*, 940—944.

Geschwind, N. and Galaburda, A. M. (1987). *Cerebral Lateralization. Biological Mechanisms, Associations, and Pathology*. Cambridge: MIT Press.

Goldman-Rakic, P. S. and Rakic, P. (1984). Experimental modification of gyral patterns. In N. Geschwind and A. M. Galaburda (eds.), *Cerebral Dominance. The Biological Foundations*. Cambridge: Harvard University Press, 179—192.

Haslam, R. H. A., Dalby, J. T., Johns, R. D. and Rademaker, A. W. (1981). Cerebral asymmetry in developmental dyslexia. *Archives of Neurology, 38*, 679—682.

Hécaen, H., De Agostini, M. and Monzon-Montes, A. (1981). Cerebral organization in left-handers. *Brain and Language, 12*, 261—284.

Henderson, V. W., Naeser, M. A., Weiner, J. M., Pieniadz, J. M. and Chui, H. C. (1984). CT criteria of hemisphere asymmetry fail to predict language laterality. *Neurology, 34*, 1086—1089.

Hier, D. B., LeMay, M., Rosenberger, P. B. and Perlo, V. P. (1978). Developmental dyslexia. Evidence for a subgroup with reversal of asymmetry. *Archives of Neurology, 35*, 90—92.

Humphreys, P., Kaufmann, W. E., Galaburda, A. M. (1990). Developmental dyslexia in women: Neuropathological findings in three cases. *Annals of Neurology, 28*, 727—738.

Humphreys, P., Rosen, G. D., Press, D. M., Sherman, G. F. and Galaburda, A. M. (1991). Freezing lesions of the developing rat brain. I. A model for cerebrocortical microgyria. *Journal of Neuropathology and Experimental Neurology, 50*, 145—160.

Hynd, G. W., Semrud-Clikeman, M., Lorys, A. R., Novey, E. S. and Eliopulos, D. (1990). Brain morphology in developmental dyslexia and attention deficit disorder/hyperactivity. *Archives of Neurology, 47*, 919—926.

Innocenti, G. M. and Berbel, P. (In press a). Analysis of an experimental cortical network: i) Architectonics of visual areas 17 and 18 after neonatal injections of ibotenic acid; similarities with human microgyria. *Journal of Neural Transplantation*.

Innocenti, G. M. and Berbel, P. (In press b). Analysis of an experimental cortical network: ii) Connections of areas 17 and 18 after neonatal injections of ibotenic acid. *Journal of Neural Transplantation*.

Kaufmann, W. E. and Galaburda, A. M. (1989). Cerebrocortical microdysgenesis in neurologically normal subjects: a histopathologic study. *Neurology, 39*, 238—244.

Mazziotta, J. C., Phelps, M. E., Carson, R. E. and Kuhl, D. E. (1982). Tomographic mapping of human cerebral metabolism: auditory stimulation. *Neurology, 32*, 921—937.

Mesulam, M-M. (1982). Slowly progressive aphasia without generalized dementia. *Annals of Neurology, 11*, 592—598.

Petersen, S. E., Fox, P. T., Posner, M. I., Mintun, M. and Raichle, M. E. (1988), Positron emission tomographic studies of the cortical anatomy of single-word processing. *Nature, 331*, 585—589.

Pfeifer, R. A. (1936). Pathologie der Hörstrahlung und der corticalen Hörsphäre. In O. Bumke and O. Förster O. (eds.), *Handbuch der Neurologie, vol. 6* Berlin: Springer, 533—626.

Rosen, G. D., Sherman, G. F. and Galaburda, A. M. (1989). Interhemispheric connections differ between symmetrical and asymmetrical brain regions. *Neuroscience, 33*, 525—533.

Rubens, A. B., Mahowald, M. W. and Hutton, J. T. (1976). Asymmetry of lateral (Sylvian) fissures in man. *Neurology, 26*, 620—624.

Rumsey, J. M., Dorwart, R., Vermess, M., Denckla, M. B., Kruesi, M. J. P. and Rapoport, J. L. (1986). Magnetic resonance imaging of brain anatomy in severe developmental dyslexia. *Archives of Neurology, 43*, 1045—1046.

Sherman, G. F., Galaburda, A. M. and Geschwind, N. (1985). Cortical anomalies in brains of New Zealand mice: a neuropathologic model of dyslexia? *Proceedings of the National Academy of Sciences (USA), 82*, 8072—8074.

Sherman, G. F., Morrison, L., Rosen, G. D., Behan, P. O. and Galaburda A. M. (1990a). Brain abnormalities in immune defective mice. *Brain Research, 532*, 25—33.

Sherman, G. F., Stone, J. S., Press, D. M., Rosen, G. D. and Galaburda, A. M. (1990b). Abnormal architecture and connections disclosed by neurofilament staining in the cerebral cortex of autoimmune mice. *Brain Research, 529*, 202—207.

Sherman, G. F., Stone, J. S., Rosen, G. D. and Galaburda, A. M. (1990c). Neocortical VIP neurons are increased in the hemisphere containing focal cerebrocortical microdysgenesis in New Zealand Black Mice. *Brain Research, 532*, 232—236.

Steingrüber, H. J. (1971). Zur Messung der Händigkeit. *Zeitschrift für Experimentelle und Angewandte Psychologie (Göttingen), 18*, 337—357.

Steinmetz, H., Fürst, G. and Freund, H.-J. (1989a). Cerebral cortical localization: application and validation of the proportional grid system in MR imaging. *Journal of Computer Assisted Tomography, 13*, 10—19.

Steinmetz, H., Fürst, G. and Freund, H.-J. (1990a). Variation of perisylvian and calcarine anatomic landmarks within stereotaxic proportional coordinates. *American Journal of Neuroradiology, 11*, 1123—1130.

Steinmetz, H., Rademacher, J., Huang, H., Hefter, H., Zilles, K., Thron, A. and Freund, H.-J. (1989b). Cerebral asymmetry: MR planimetry of the human planum temporale. *Journal of Computer Assisted Tomography, 13*, 996—1005.

Steinmetz, H., Rademacher, J., Jäncke, L., Huang, Y., Thron, A. and Zilles, K. (1990b). Total surface of temporoparietal intrasylvian cortex: diverging left-right asymmetries. *Brain and Language, 39*, 357—372.

Steinmetz, H., Volkmann, J., Jäncke, L. and Freund, H.-J. (1991). Anatomical left-right asymmetry of language-related temporal cortex is different in left- and right-handers. *Annals of Neurology, 29*, 315—319.

Yeni-Komshian, G. H. and Benson, D. A. (1976). Anatomical study of cerebral asymmetry in the temporal lobe of humans, chimpanzees, and rhesus monkeys. *Science, 192*, 387—389.

consistencies between neurolinguistic theory as articulated by Geschwind (1974; 1984) and his colleagues (Geschwind and Galaburda, 1985a, 1985b, 1985c; Geschwind and Levitsky, 1968) and the results of the neuroimaging studies.

LANGUAGE AND CEREBRAL ASYMMETRIES

In the past 20 years, neuroimaging and postmortem studies have begun to provide more direct evidence implicating neuropathological structures in dyslexia. With the advent of computed tomography (CT) scanning and magnetic resonance imaging (MRI), it is possible to examine directly deviations in brain structure in children with dyslexia. Using neuroimaging techniques to examine deviations in brain morphology represents an extension of the increasing evidence documenting reliable patterns of human brain asymmetry. Numerous patterns of normal brain asymmetries have been identified. For example, Weinberger, Luchins, Morihisa, and Wyatt (1982) and LeMay (1976) demonstrated in normals that the volume of the right frontal region exceeds the left in 75% of the brains they examined. Furthermore, the difference in asymmetry appears in the 20th week of fetal development (Witelson and Pallie, 1973). Left greater than right asymmetries have also been noted in the anterior speech region (Falzi, Perrone and Vignolo, 1982), in the left auditory cortex (Galaburda and Sanides, 1980), and in the posterior thalamus (Eidelberg and Galaburda, 1982). Though each of these asymmetries is considered vital to language development (Campbell and Whitaker, 1986), asymmetries in the central language area appear to be especially significant.

Based on the work of Flechsig (1908) and Von Economo and Horn (1930), Geschwind and Levitsky (1968) documented that in 100 normal adult brains they studied, 65% had larger left than right planum temporale. By contrast, only 11% had larger right than left plana. Furthermore, they reported that the left planum temporale is about one-third longer than the right. Similar studies by other investigators documented these findings in both adult and infant brains (Kopp, Michel, Carrier, Biron, and Duvillard, 1977; Rubens, Mahuwald, and Hutton, 1976; Teszner, Tzavaras, Gruner, and Hecaen, 1972; Wada, Clarke, and Hamm, 1975; Witelson and Pallie, 1973). Because the left temporal cortex is known to be associated with language, these findings were interpreted as reflecting a natural neurobiological substrata important to language.

Geschwind (1974, 1984) and Geschwind and Galaburda (1985a, 1985b, 1985c) further argue that natural asymmetries in brain morphology are associated with language and with language-based disorders, such as dyslexia. There is considerable support for their position. Whereas two thirds of normal brains show a left greater than right posterior asymmetry, only 10% to 50% of dyslexic brains show this pattern (Hier, LeMay, Rosenberger, and Perlo, 1978; Haslam, Dalby, Johns, Rademeker, 1981; Rumsey, *et al.*, 1986). Cytoarchitectonic studies reveal a higher-than-normal incidence of plana symmetry and focal dysplasias involving the left frontal, left perisylvian, and right frontal regions (Galaburda and Kemper, 1979; Galaburda *et al.*, 1985).

The work of Geschwind and others generally supports the notion that deviations in normal patterns of brain asymmetry are meaningfully associated with developmental dyslexia. Despite accumulating evidence that such a connection exists, specific measures of deviations have, until recently, been lacking. Part of the problem has been technical. Introduced in 1973, CT scanning has proven its clinical value in identifying pathologic problems, such as changes in tissue density, enlarged ventricular size, midline shifts, and vascular abnormalities. However, CT has not been consistently useful in evaluating disorders of developmental origin such as nonspecific mental retardation (Lingam *et al.*, 1982; Moeschler, Bennett, and Cromwell, 1981). However, neurolinguistic theory predicts that gross structural deviations are not correlated with the often subtle behavioral manifestations of dyslexia; rather, deviations in patterns of normal asymmetry appear to be correlated with dyslexia. In this context, then, brain imaging studies may help link deviant patterns of brain asymmetry with the behavioral manifestations of dyslexia.

BRAIN IMAGING IN DYSLEXIA: METHODOLOGICAL ISSUES

In the past decade, nine neuroimaging studies of dyslexic subjects have been reported. These studies include more than 200 children and adults with severe reading and learning problems. Their results are summarized by Hynd and Semrud-Clikeman (1989b). Some general comments are helpful before reviewing the results of these studies. First, only four of the nine used a control population for comparison. In studies which included control subjects, the ratio of controls to dyslexics ranged from 0.25:1 (Leisman and Ashkenazi, 1980) to .31:1 (Haslam *et al.*, 1981) to 5.78:1 (Parkins, Roberts, Reinarz, and Varney, 1987) to 11.74:1 (LeMay, 1981). Thus, in studies contrasting deviations in the asymmetry of dyslexics' brains, only the LeMay and Parkins *et al.* studies included sufficient controls to make such a comparison meaningful. Moreover, criteria for "control" were neither consistent nor relevant. For example, one control group was referred for headaches, and it is not known whether they had normal patterns of brain morphology. Also, none of the studies included psychometric data for the controls; thus it cannot be known whether these subjects were free of other behavioral, neurological, or psychiatric disorders.

Second, the age range of the subjects may be a relevant factor in terms of the nature of the dyslexia. It is possible, but difficult, to document whether the younger subjects used in some of these studies (e.g., Haslam *et al.*, 1981) represent as severe a manifestation of reading disability as was found in the adults examined (Rumsey *et al.*, 1986; Parkins *et al.*, 1987). Also, as Morris, Blashfield, and Satz (1986) point out, there may be a Development x Dyslexia Subtype interaction resulting in different neuropsychological subtypes in the older subjects.

Handedness of children and adults with developmental dyslexia has resulted in a large body of conflicting evidence (Corballis and Beale, 1976; Kinsbourne and Hiscock, 1981). With the exceptions of Leisman and Ashkenazi (1980) and Denckla, LeMay, and Chapman (1985), handedness is typically reported in these studies. However, only the Rumsey *et al.* (1986) study cites a specific measure a handedness. Moreover, all of these studies treat handedness as a unifactorial discontinuous variable. As Coren, Porac, and Duncan (1979) point out, handedness is a multifactorial variable and handedness and laterality data should be treated as a continuous variable.

Although some of these studies did not include subjects who were left-handed (e.g., Haslam *et al.*, 1981), those which did suggest that left handers are over-represented in these subjects. For example, Hier et al. (1978) reported that 6 of 24 subjects (25%) were left-handed; LeMay (1981) reported 22.2%; Rosenberger and Hier (1980) reported 15.1%; and Parkins *et al.* (1987) reported 20.5%. Assuming that 8—10% of the population is left-handed (Hardyck, Petrinovitch, and Goldman, 1976), the twofold increase reported in these neuroimaging studies suggests possible alternations from normal patterns of lateral organization (Geschwind and Behan, 1982).

To summarize, it appears that some of the studies are so poorly controlled or reported (e.g., Leisman and Ashkenazi, 1980; LeMay, 1981) that the results do not make important contributions to the literature. The Denckla *et al.* (1985), Hier *et al.* (1978) and Rosenberger and Hier (1980) studies appear to provide adequate diagnostic or clinical information, but in each case, essential data are omitted. In the Hier *et al.* (1978) study, Full Scale IQ scores are not reported; in the Denckla *et al.* (1985) and Rosenberger and Hier (1980) studies, adequate achievement data are not provided.

Several of the studies report sufficient diagnostic details and supporting data regarding both levels of general ability and achievement deficits in reading. Reasonable assurance exists as to the inclusion of subjects who evidence at least average intellectual ability, have a significant discrepancy in reading achievement, and are free from other behavioral, neurological, or psychiatric disorders. The studies of Haslam *et al.* (1981), Parkins *et al.* (1987), and Rumsey *et al.* (1986) offer a greater degree of confidence in terms of the populations studied. With these considerations in mind, it is appropriate to consider in detail the findings of the CT/MRI studies.

BRAIN IMAGING IN DYSLEXIA: CT/MRI FINDINGS

It is important to keep in mind that in the studies reported here, the scans were evaluated for obvious neurostructural abnormalities as well as for deviations in normal patterns of left greater than right parieto-occipital asymmetry. Based on the neuro-biological theory of Geschwind (1974; 1984) Geschwind and Behan (1982) and Geschwind and Levitsky (1968), the latter is correlated with unique neurolinguistic processes including those evidenced in reading and writing disabilities.

Despite the importance of the left planum temporale to lateralized language processes and in neurological conceptualizations of dyslexia (Chui and Damasio, 1980; Geschwind and Levitsky, 1968; Wada *et al.*, 1975; Witelson and Pallie, 1973) only one of the eight studies (Parkins *et al.* 1987) specifies the CT slice used. Parkins *et al.* (1987) selected a CT slice that corresponded most closely to Slice SM (Naeser and Hayward, 1978). This slice tranverses the region of the planum temporale, and it may produce the highest interrater reliability of clinical judgments regarding asymmetries (Pieniadz, Naeser, Koff, and Levine, 1983).

In a study by Pieniadz and Naeser (1984) Slice SM was the only one in which derived CT scan occipital length measurements correlated significantly with planum temporale length measurements made postmortem. In fact, Slice SM was the only one of six CT slices examined that correlated with postmortem measurements. In studies in which other slices may have been used to judge asymmetries, there exists no documentation that CT asymmetries correlate to actual brain morphology. Thus, even where standard asymmetry indexes were used, the resulting measurements might not correlate with true structural deviations.

A consistent finding in six of eight of these studies is that in nonconsecutively diagnosed dyslexics varying in age from 8 years to over 57 years, significantly less L > R asymmetry is present, and there is increased symmetry, or, to a lesser extent, reversed R > L parieto-occiptal asymmetry. There are two studies that fail to report this finding (Denckla *et al.*, 1985; Parkins *et al.*, 1987). In one case (Denckla *et al.*, 1985) cerebral asymmetries were not appraised, and in the other (Parkins *et al.*, 1987), this finding was observed only in left-handed dyslexics.

Most of these studies examined only parietooccipital asymmetries and LeMay (1976) found in her control population that 67% evidenced L > R width patterns. The same pattern of asymmetry was noted to be present in only 33.3% of dyslexic subjects in the Hier *et al.* (1978) study and in 46% of the dyslexics in the Haslam *et al.* (1981) study. Leisman and

Ashkenazi (1980) reported that seven of the dyslexics had the reversed (R > L) pattern, while one had equivalent cerebral hemispheres. The degree of reversed cerebral asymmetry in three studies for which comparable data are reported (Hier *et al.*, 1978; Haslam *et al.*, 1981; Leisman and Ashkenazi, 1980) averages 19.67%, just slightly more than the 13.3% reported by LeMay (1976). Compared to this, and perhaps adding strength to the argument that symmetry (Haslam *et al.*, 1981) or reversed asymmetry (Hier *et al.*, 1978; Rosenberger and Hier, 1980) is more often found in the brains of dyslexics, is the fact that across four studies (Haslam *et al.*, 1981; Hier *et al.*, 1978; Leisman and Ashkenazi, 1980; Rumsey *et al.*, 1986) an average of 58% of the CT scans were determined to be symmetrical in the parietooccipital region among the dyslexics. This high percentage of dyslexic brains showing equivalent or symmetrical parietooccipital CT regions is considerably greater than the 13.3% LeMay (1976) reported originally or the 20.5% she reported later (LeMay, 1981).

Only two studies reported frontal asymmetries in their developmental dyslexics (Haslam *et al.*, 1981; Parkins *et al.*, 1987) and it appears that Denckla *et al.* (1985) used Evans' index (Evans, 1942; Synek, Reuben and DuBoulay, 1976) to examine frontal horn abnormalities. The data derived from Denckla *et al's.*, (1985) study were not reported, although the authors noted that Evans' ratio fell within the normal range for children with learning disablilities, including those with the right hemisyndrome. drome.

In the Haslam *et al.* (1981) study, there do not appear to be very significant differences in frontal asymmetry between the developmental dyslexics and the control subjects. There were, however, proportionately more dyslexic children with equivalent frontal hemispheres than would be expected from LeMay's (1976) earlier normative findings. Because the original data are not provided, however, it is impossible to determine if this is a statistically significant finding. Parkins *et al.*, (1987) analyzed their data regarding frontal measurements and reported that for the developmental dyslexics, no significant differences existed with respect to previously collected (Chui and Damasio, 1980) normative data on any frontal measure.

Consequently, it appears that developmental dyslexics may have an increased incidence of posterior symmetry (Haslam *et al.*, 1981; Rumsey *et al.*, 1986) or, in dyslexics with serious expressive language delay (as measured by history and verbal IQ), perhaps a higher incidence of reversed parietooccipital asymmetry (Hier *et al.*, 1978; Leisman and Ashkenazi, 1980; LeMay, 1981; Rosenberger and Hier, 1980). Although these suggest posterior symmetry and reversed parietooccipital asymmetry, they clearly are at variance with the findings recently reported by Parkins *et al.* (1987) who examined 44 CT scans of developmental dyslexic adults.

Parkins *et al.* (1987) found it was only among left-handed dyslexics that there were proportionately fewer cases of L > R parietooccipital asymmetry; this finding was particularly significant regarding the length measurement. Thus, in the sample of adults examined by Parkins *et al.* (1987) the findings of less posterior asymmetry is only relevant in left-handed dyslexics.

There seems to be some agreement that dyslexics evidence some degree of symmetry of the posterior cortex, but the various studies differ with respect to the influence of handedness, with the Parkins *et al.* (1987) study standing alone in suggesting that this effect is only observed in left-handed developmental dyslexics.

Although the possible long-term developmental interactions between severity of dyslexia, cognitive ability, handedness, and cerebral asymmetries are unknown, it may be postulated that among young right-handed dyslexics (<8–25 years) symmetry or an increased incidence of reversed asymmetry characterizes some subjects. Furthermore, should interactions exist between handedness and cerebral asymmetries among dyslexics, only the Parkins *et al.* (1987) study suggests that this may be a consideration.

Unfortunately the CT/MRI studies suffer from serious methodological flaws which may be contributing to the discordant findings reported by the authors. Specifically, more adequate reporting of population and methodological variables should have been provided. These included achievement and handedness data, CT/MRI transaxial slices used, intracranial measurements, relations between detailed linguistic or reading parameters and brain morphology. Hynd and Semrud-Clikeman (1989a, 1989b) provide a detailed review of these concerns.

In addition, certain technical problems emerge from this review. These include (a) the failure of some studies to specify the type or generation of CT scanner used (Haslam *et al.*, 1981; Hier *et al.*, 1978; Liesman and Ashkenazi, 1980; LeMay, 1981); (b) the lack of specifics regarding the CT/MRI scan sections examined (Leisman and Ashkenazi, 1980; LeMay, 1981, Rumsey *et al.*, 1986); and (c) the use of nonmetric clinical procedures in judging presence/absence of normal patterns of asymmetry or symmetry in some studies (Leisman and Ashkenazi, 1980; Rumsey *et al.*, 1986). The latter precludes comparing their relative importance to other studies as well as examining for possible relations with levels of achievement or IQ variables in their subjects.

UNIVERSITY OF GEORGIA BRAIN IMAGING STUDIES

Primarily because of these methodological flaws, CT/MRI procedures have provided only limited evidence that alterations in normal patterns of brain asymmetry in the region of the left planum temporale and parietooccipital cortex may correlate with the behaviorally defined syndrome of developmental dyslexia. In a recent study, Hynd *et al.* (1990) investigated possible differences in patterns of brain asymmetry between children with a diagnosis of dyslexia, a clinic control group of children with Attention Deficit Disorder with Hyperactivity (ADD/H), and normal control subjects. This study addressed some of the methodological issues identified earlier. First, the authors used a carefully devised neuropsychological battery which reliably diagnosed dyslexia and which differentiated normal and dyslexic subjects (Table 1). Second, they used precise morphometric measures to assess regional variations in brain structure.

Table 1. Means and standard deviations on the dependent measures for all groups

Dependent variable	Dyslexic	ADD/H	Normal
Age	118.9 (24.55)	120.6 (40.43)	141.20 (24.07)
FSIQ	108 (8.68)	109.3 (12.27)	125.90 (10.91)
Verbal comp.	11.65 (2.18)	11.29 (2.87)	14.05 (1.65)
Word attack	73.8 (14.91)	96.30 (16.47)	115.60 (9.97)
Passage comp.	75.0 (17.17)	99.40 (10.78)	112.30 (12.34)
PPVT-R	100.7 (10.93)	101.80 (16.42)	122.50 (12.34)
Boston naming	39.2 (7.96)	41.70 (7.44)	52.20 (5.20)
RAN (errors)	3.0 (2.83)	0.50 (1.26)	0.00 (0.00)
RAN (time)	198.8 (84.69)	160.10 (65.21)	118.40 (31.13)
RAS (errors)	1.5 (1.90)	0.50 (0.71)	0.20 (0.63)
RAS (time)	108.2 (36.44)	99.60 (30.42)	54.00 (47.76)
VMI	94.5 (13.00)	94.00 (15.24)	109.50 (7.62)

Parentheses denote standard deviation.

Table 2 and Figure 1 summarize the results of the brain morphology measures for each group. Figure 1 shows reversed (L < R) or symmetrical plana temporale length in the dyslexic subjects while the normal and ADD/H children had the expected pattern of L > R plana length. Additionally, the dyslexic and ADD/H samples showed smaller insular region length bilaterally as well as symmetrical frontal regions (Figures 2, 3).

As predicted, there was a significant relationship between the study's neurolinguistic measures and selected brain measurements. The former include word attack and passage comprehension subtests and automatized and confrontation naming tasks. Children with lower scores on these tasks showed reversed asymmetry or symmetrical measures on the length of the plana temporale, the insular region, and the frontal areas. Because of its significant findings and because it was specifically designed to investigate

Table 2. Means and standard deviations for brain morphology measures for three groups

Measure	Dyslexics	ADD/H	Normal
Total area	144.05 (8.11)	143.41 (15.76)	144.355 (9.12)
Left frontal area	18.44 (1.53)	18.93 (2.06)	18.95 (2.56)
Right frontal area	19.304 (2.75)	19.71 (1.65)	20.49 (2.93)
Left plana length	1.20 (0.41)	1.41 (0.212)	1.52 (0.35)
Right plana length	1.32 (0.374)	1.20 (0.298)	1.34 (0.386)
Left insular length	4.52 (0.88)	4.8 (0.535)	5.15 (0.5798)
Right insular length	4.36 (0.753)	4.64 (0.657)	5.18 (0.56)
Left frontal width	5.23 (0.195)	5.3 (0.313)	5.42 (0.257)
Right frontal width	5.23 (0.183)	5.39 (0.304)	5.59 (0.288)

Parentheses denote standard deviation

possible relationships between brain morphology and the neurolinguistic deficits found in dyslexia, the study's methodologies are worth reviewing.

Diagnostic Procedures

Subjects were divided into three groups. There were 10 subjects with diagnosed dyslexia, 10 with ADD/H, and 10 normal controls. Each subject was administered a day-long comprehensive neuropsychological battery. This battery included a test of general intellectual ability, a reading

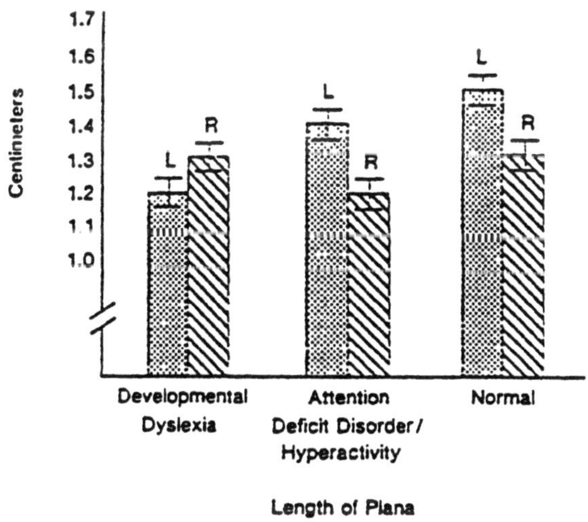

Fig. 1. Group and hemispheric differences in the length of the plana region of interest measurements. L indicates left; R, right. Reprinted with permission from Hynd *et al.* (1990).

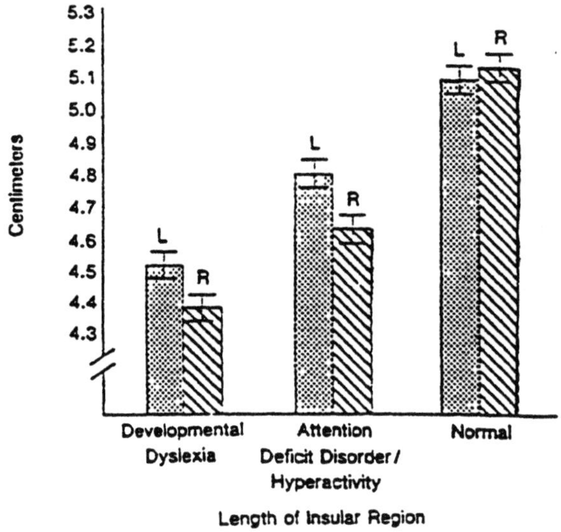

Fig. 2. Group and hemispheric differences in the length of the insular region of interest measurements. L indicates left, R, right. Reprinted with permission from Hynd *et al.* (1990).

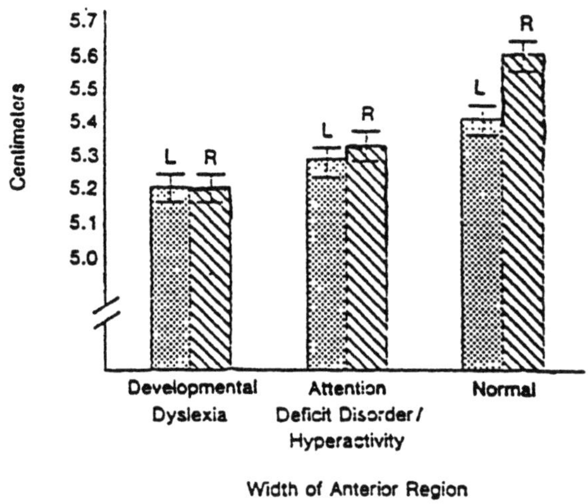

Fig. 3. Group and hemispheric differences in the width of the anterior region of interest measurements. L indicates left; R, right. Reprinted with permission from Hynd *et al.* (1990).

test, various neuropsychological measures, a test of handedness, and a family history of autoimmune disease. Behavioral information was obtained through parent interview and through parent and teacher rating scales.

Diagnostic criteria for dyslexia included at least normal Full Scale IQ on the WISC-R, a positive family history of learning problems, personal history of reading disabilities, reading achievement greater than or equal to 20 standard score points below FSIO on *both* the Word Attack and Passage Comprehension subtest of the WRMT-R, and no reported symptoms of hyperactivity.

MRI Protocol

MRI scanning was conducted on all subjects using a 0.6-T Technicare Scanner (Health Images; Atlanta, Ga.). Sequential T1, sagittal, and axial planes were obtained. The protocol included fifteen 7.5 mm sagittal planes (TR = 690; TE = 32) and eleven 5 mm axial planes (TR = 500, TE = 32) was used. Region of interest measurements were obtained using the Technicare ROI Measurement software system.

Postmortem studies document that the axial slice transversing the region of the planum temporale (including, in part, the supramarginal and angular gyri) is the only slice that correlated significantly with morphological measurements (Pieniadz and Naeser, 1984). Consequently, an axial slice of this region of interest (ROI) was selected for analysis. ROI measurements were made for the width and area of the left and right anterior (from a line drawn horizontally across the posterior tip of the genu) and posterior (from a line drawn horizontally across the posterior tip of the splenium) regions; the length of the left and right insular regions; and for total brain area.

Recognizing the significant variability in brain morphologic findings and that some of the ROI may not be easily judged (Witelson, 1982), 10 scans were randomly selected and an independent measure obtained for each ROI. The initial measurements were made by an experienced radiological technician specifically trained to identify the ROI. The reliability check was completed by a pediatric neuropsychologist with expertise in developmental neuroanatomy. Reliability coefficients were excellent (x = 0.95) across 13 ROI measurements.

Significant differences appeared in general intellectual ability (normal children higher than those with either dyslexia or ADD/H), in handedness (more dyslexics were left handed), and in the number and kinds of codiagnoses (ADD/H had more codiagnoses).

There were no significant differences across ages or in total brain areas among the three groups of subjects. It seems reasonable to assume, therefore, that differences in patterns of hemispheric asymmetry or symmetry are associated with regional variations in neurological development and not with gross differences in brain morphology. Significant differences in regional variations are reported in anterior-width measurements. Whereas normals evidenced the expected pattern of left less than right asymmetry, both dyslexic and ADD/H children had bilaterally smaller anterior cortexes.

The length of the insular region also differed significantly between groups. Dyslexic children had shorter insular regions bilaterally than either the normal or the ADD/H subjects. The dyslexic group also differed significantly from the normal group in left planum temporale length. It was also reported that 90% of the dyslexic children had either symmetry or reversed asymmetry (L < R) of plana length. Assuming that 30% L < R plana length is normal, the 90% incidence in dyslexic children represents a very significant departure from normal patterns of differential brain maturation.

Results of this study document the uniqueness of an increased incidence of L < R plana length symmetry/reversed asymmetry in the brains of dyslexic children. That there were no significant differences in total brain area in the dyslexic, ADD/H, and normal subjects suggests that the regional variation in brain morphology is due to a more specific deviation in brain ontogeny. The fact that dyslexics consistently showed smaller areas (left planum, bilateral insular regions, and right anterior region) known to be implicated in language is seen as further support for deviations in normal patterns of brain development.

The finding that 70% of normal and ADD/H children had left greater than right asymmetry in the plana supports similar studies using CT/MRI (LeMay, 1981; Rumsey *et al.*, 1986; Hynd and Semrud-Clikeman, 1989b) and postmortem data (Geschwind and Levitsky, 1968; Witelson and Pallie, 1973). Furthermore, the 90% incidence of L < R in the dyslexics in the length of the planum temporale is a threefold increase over normal base rates. Because the dyslexic subjects and normal subjects did not differ significantly in right plana length (1.32 cm vs 1.34 cm, respectively) but did in left plana length (1.20 cm vs 1.52 cm, respectively) it seems that some deviation in corticogenesis preferentially affects the left planum temporale during development. This conclusion would be consistent with that of some authors (e.g., Witelson, 1982) but it is at odds with Galaburda, Corsiglia, Rosen, and Sherman (1987) who propose that the right plana is preferentially enhanced during fetal development. Clearly, further imaging and postmortem studies are needed to address this issue.

The finding of a bilaterally smaller insular region in dyslexia is also of interest, because the left insular region has been associated with language disturbance. The relative importance of the insular region in dyslexia was established in positron emission tomography studies of regional cerebral glucose metabolism (rCMRglc) in which dyslexics showed bilaterally decreased levels of rCMRglc during reading (Gross-Glenn, *et al.*, 1986). It may be that the bilaterally smaller regions found in dyslexics in this study correlate with the hypometabolic activity of the insular region observed in the positron emission tomography study.

Significantly smaller anterior-width measurements were also observed in the dyslexic subjects. Both dyslexic and ADD/H subjects lacked normal left less than right asymmetry of the anterior region; both groups also had significantly smaller right anterior-width measurements than did normal control children. That dyslexics showed consistently small regions that are related to language is considered further evidence suggesting that there is some deviation in normal patterns of brain development in children with dyslexia.

The study by Hynd *et al.* (1990) makes two relevant contributions. First, it corroborates previous findings from postmortem and CT studies already demonstrating a relationship between brain morphology and language. And second, it establishes a foundation for examining the relationship between variations in brain morphology and measures of neurolinguistic functioning. This will be discussed in the next section.

Neurolinguistic Relationships

Relationships between brain morphology measures and reading and naming tasks are also illuminating. For example, in a further analysis of the Hynd *et al.* (1990) data, Semrud-Clikeman, Hynd, Novey, and Eliopulos (in press) reported a significant interaction between anterior-width measurements and passage comprehension. Dyslexic subjects (with smaller anterior regions) were found to perform significantly poorer than subjects with normal asymmetry patterns. Bilateral hypoperfusion (Lou, Henriksen, and Bruhn, 1984, 1989) and increased cytoarchitectonic anomalies have also been reported in the frontal regions (Galaburda *et al.*, 1985). These data suggest that children with dyslexia may have insufficient substrata available for processing.

Patterns of asymmetry may also be related to specific language tasks. For example, Semrud-Clikeman *et al.* (in press) reported that when the asymmetry of the anterior region was reversed, all groups performed poorer on a test measuring word attack skills. Passage comprehension was not affected by reversed asymmetry. Figure 4 illustrates the magnitude of this effect.

Due to insufficient group size, it was impossible to conduct a plana asymmetry x group x neuropsychological ANOVA. Instead, this analysis was conducted on a dichotomized distribution of subjects. In this distribution, 15 subjects were assigned to each group based on whether their left or right plana was longer. Significant differences between these two groups

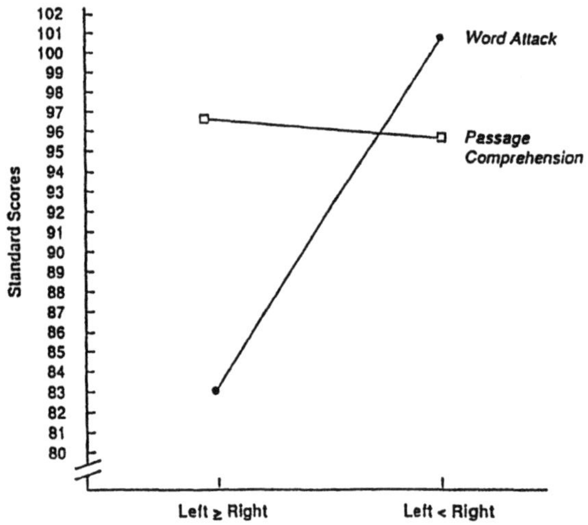

Fig. 4. Interaction between frontal area asymmetry and performance on word attack and passage comprehension measures. Reprinted with permission from Semrud-Clikeman *et al.* (in press).

were found on all neuropsychological measures except for IQ and Total Time on the Rapid Naming Test (Semrud-Clikeman *et al.*, in press).

Consistent differences in insular region length and left planum temporale area and deficient performance on naming and reading tests in the dyslexic subjects leads to speculation as to the relationship between these areas and specific language abilities (Geschwind and Galaburda, 1985a, 1985b, 1985c; Hynd and Semrud-Clikemen, 1989a, 1989b). In the case of true developmental dyslexia, the ability to encode letters, numbers, colors, and letter-sound associations may be inhibited by morphological differences present from birth; however, it is not yet clear whether poorer neurolinguistic development is due to diminished regional size or to reversed asymmetry/symmetry in specific regions, in this case, the anterior region, the planum temporale, and the insular cortex. Consistent with Hier *et al.* (1978) and Rosenberger and Hier (1980), it is hypothesized that developmental differences in brain morphology may place the child "at risk" for dyslexia, but that the probability of dyslexia manifesting itself increases when these pathoanatomic differences are present in several regions. It may be, therefore, that the important variables are the *pattern* and *extent* of the asymmetry/symmetry rather than the specific deviation itself. For example, when reversed asymmetry of the planum temporale is the only deviation, there may be little or no significant interference with reading performance. It must be kept in mind that approximately 30% of *normal* brains show symmetry or reversed asymmetry in the central-posterior region (Geschwind and Levitsky, 1968; Hier *et al.*, 1990). Differential effects of neurolinguistic functioning based on patterns of deviations in brain morphology would also explain why some children experience difficulties in reading and naming while overall intelligence, visual-spatial skills, or receptive language abilities may remain relatively intact.

CONCLUSION

The overview provided in this article suggests several conclusions. First, it is evident that neuroimaging procedures may provide important data in documenting deviations in normal patterns of brain asymmetry, and that these deviations may be linked to the behavioral manifestations of developmental dyslexia. Second, more recent studies indicate that deviations in normal patterns of frontal and insular morphology may also characterize the brains of dyslexics (Hynd *et al.*, 1990; Semrud-Clikeman *et al.*, in press). Third, the two most recent studies fail to demonstrate a link between patterns of plana asymmetry-symmetry and handedness in dyslexia (Hynd *et al.*, 1990; Larsen, Høien, Lundberg, and Odegaard, 1990). Finally, there are many conceptual and technical issues that remain unresolved.

Neuroimaging procedures are increasingly being employed in evaluating important theoretical issues in childhood developmental disorders such as dyslexia, Attention-Deficit Hyperactivity Disorder, and Autism (Kuperman *et al.*, 1990). By employing new MRI protocols allowing for whole brain imaging (Filipek *et al.*, 1989) and by examining the topography of other brain regions that may also be implicated in dyslexia, such as the parietal opercular region (Steinmetz, Uberling, Huang, and Kahn, 1990) our knowledge as to the neuroanatomical basis of dyslexia may be significantly enhanced in the next decade.

Note: This article summarizes a program of research conducted at the University of Georgia. As such, some of the content of this article was abstracted with permission from Hynd and Semrud-Clikeman (1989a, 1989b), Hynd *et al.* (1990), and Semrud-Clikeman *et al.* (in press).

ACKNOWLEDGEMENT

The research conducted by the senior author and discussed in this article was supported in part by grants from the RGK and Donald D. Hammill Foundations. The support from these Foundations is gratefully acknowledged.

Requests for reprints should be addressed to George W. Hynd, Center for Clinical and Developmental Neuropsychology, EXC-Aderhold Hall, University of Georgia, Athens, Georgia, 30602.

REFERENCES

Campbell, S., and Whitaker, H. (1986). Cortical maturation and developmental neurolinguistics. In J. E. Obrzut and G. W. Hynd (eds.), *Child Neuropsychology: Theory and Research* Vol. 1, pp. 55—72). New York: Academic Press.

Chui, H. C., and Damasio, A. R. (1980). Human cerebral asymmetries evaluated by computerized tomography. *Journal of Neurology, Neurosurgery, and Psychiatry, 43*, 873—878.

Corballis, M. C., and Beale, I. C. (1976). *The Psychology of Left and Right.* Hillsdale, NJ: Erlbaum.

Coren, S., Porac, C., and Duncan, P. (1979). A behaviorally validated self-report inventory to assess four types of lateral preference. *Journal of Clinical Neuropsychology, 1*, 33—64.

Denckla, M. B., LeMay, M., and Chapman, C. A. (1985). Few CT scan abnormalities found even in neurologically impaired learning disabled children. *Journal of Learning Disabilities, 18*, 132—135.

Eidelberg, D., and Galabruda, A. M. (1982). Symmetry and asymmetry in the human posterior thalamus: I Cytoarchitectonic analysis in normal persons. *Archives of Neurology, 39*, 325—332.

Evans, W. A. (1942). An encephalographic ratio for estimating ventricular enlargement and cerebral atrophy. *Archives of Neurology, 47*, 931—937.

Falzi, G., Perrone, P., and Vignolo, L. A. (1982). Right-left asymmetry in anterior speech region. *Archives of Neurology, 39*, 239—240.

Filipek, P. A., Kennedy, D. N., Caviness, V. S., Rossnick, S. L., Spraggins, T. A., Starewicz, P. M. (1989). Magnetic resonance imaging-based brain morphology: Development and application to normal subjects. *Annals of Neurology, 25*, 61—67.

Fleschig, P. (1908). *Zentrablatt Neurologie-Psychiatrie, 27*, 50.

Galaburda, A. M., and Kemper, T. L. (1979). Cytoarchitectonic abnormalities in developmental dyslexia: a case study. *Annals of Neurology, 6*, 94—100.

Galaburda, A., and Sanides, F. (1980). Cytoarchitectonic organization of the human auditory cortex. *Journal of Comparative Neurology, 190*, 597—610.

Galaburda, A. M., Sherman, G. F., Rosen, G. D., Aboitiz, F., Geschwind, N. (1985). Developmental dyslexia: Four consecutive patients with cortical abnormalities. *Annuals of Neurology, 18*, 222—233.

Galaburda, A. M., Corsiglia, J., Rosen, G. D., and Sherman, G. F. (1987). Planum temporale asymmetry, reappraisal since Geschwind and Levitsky. *Neuropsychologia, 25*, 853—868.

Geschwind, N. (1974). The development of the brain and the evolution of language. In N. Geschwind (eds.), *Selected Papers on Language and the Brain.* Dordrecht, The Netherlands: D. Reidel.

Geschwind, N. (1984). Cerebral dominance in biological perspective. *Neuropsychologia, 22*, 675—683.

Geschwind, N., and Behan, P. O. (1982). Left handedness: Association with immune disease, migraine, and developmental learning disorders. *Proceedings of the National Academy of Sciences, 79*, 5097—5100.

Geschwind, N., and Galaburda, A. M. (1985a). Cerebral lateralization: Biological mechanisms, associations, and pathology: I. A hypothesis and a program for research. *Archives of Neurology, 42*, 428—459.

Geschwind, N., and Galaburda, A. M. (1985b). Cerebral lateralization: Biological mechanisms, associations, and pathology: II. A hypothesis and a program for research. *Archives of Neurology, 42,* 521–552.

Geschwind, N., and Galaburda, A. M. (1985c). Cerebral lateralization: Biological mechanisms, associations, and pathology: III. A hypothesis and a program for research. *Archives of Neurology, 42,* 634–654.

Geschwind, N., and Levitsky, W. (1968). Human brain: Left-right asymmetries in temporal speech region. *Science, 161,* 186–187.

Golden, G. S. (1982). Neurobiological correlates of learning disabilities. *Annals of Neurology, 12,* 409–418.

Gross-Glenn, K., Duara, R., Yoshii, F., Baker, W. W., Chang, J. Y., Apicella, A., Boothe, T., and Lubs, H. A. (1986). PET-scan studies during reading in dyslexic and non-dyslexic adults [abstract], *Neuroscience, 24,* 371.

Hardyck, C., Petrinovitch, L. F., and Goldman, R. (1976). Left handedness and cognitive deficit. *Cortex, 12,* 266–278.

Harris, T. L., and Hodges, R. E. (eds.). (1981). *A Dictionary of Reading and Related Terms.* Newark, NJ: International Reading Association.

Haslam, R. H., Dalby, J. T., Johns, R. D., and Rademaker, A. W. (1981). Cerebral asymmetry in developmental dyslexia. *Archives of Neurology, 38,* 679–682.

Hier, D. B., LeMay, M. Rosenberger, P. B., and Perlo, V. P. (1978). Developmental dyslexia: Evidence for a subgroup with a reversal of cerebral asymmetry. *Archives of Neurology, 35,* 90–92.

Hynd, G. W., and Semrud-Clikeman, M. (1989a). Dyslexia and neurodevelopmental pathology: Relationships to cognition, intelligence and reading skill acquisition. *Journal of Learning Disabilities, 22,* 204–216.

Hynd, G. W., and Semrud-Clikeman, M. (1989b). Dyslexia and brain morphology. *Psychological Bulletin, 106,* 447–482.

Hynd, G. W., Semrud-Clikeman, M.. Lorys, A. R., Novey, E. S., and Eliopulos, D. (1990). Brain morphology in developmental dyslexia and attention deficit disorder/hyperactivity. *Archives of Neurology, 47,* 919–926.

Kinsbourne, M., and Hiscock, M. (1981). Cerebral lateralization and cognitive development: Conceptual and methodological issues. In G. W. Hynd and J. E. Obrzut (eds.), *Neuropsychological Assessment and the School-Age Child: Issues and Procedures* (pp. 125–166). New York: Grune and Stratton.

Kopp, N., Michel, F., Carrier, H., Biron, A., and Duvillard, P. (1977). Etude de certaines asymetries hemispheriques du cerveau humain. *Journal of the Neurological Sciences, 34,* 349–363.

Kuperman, S., Gaffney, G. R., Hamden-Allen, G., Preston, D. F., and Venkatesh, L. (1990). Neuroimaging in child and adolescent psychiatry. *Journal of the American Academy of Child and Adolescent Psychiatry, 29,* 159–172.

Larsen, J. P., Høien, T., Lundberg, I., and Odegaard, H. (1990). MRI evaluation of the size and symmetry of the planum temporale in adolescents with developmental dyslexia. *Brain and Language, 39,* 289–301.

Leisman, G., and Ashkenazi, M. (1980). Aetiological factors in dyslexia: IV. Cerebral hemispheres are functionally equivalent. *Neuroscience, 11,* 157–164.

LeMay, M. (1976). Morphological cerebral asymmetries of modern man, fossil man, and nonhuman primates. *Annals of the New York Academy of Science, 280,* 349–366.

LeMay, M. (1981). Are there radiological changes in the brains of individuals with dyslexia? *Bulletin of the Orton Society, 31,* 135–141.

Lingam, S., Read, S., Holland, I. M., Wilson, J., Brett, E. M., and Hoare, R. D. (1982). Value of computerized tomography in children with non-specific mental subnormality. *Archives of Disease in Childhood, 57,* 381–383.

Lou, H. C., Henriksen, L., and Bruhn, P. (1984). Focal cerebral hypoperfusion in children with dysphasia and/or attention deficit disorder. *Archives of Neurology, 41*, 852—829.

Lou, H. C., Henriksen, L., and Bruhn, P. (1989). Striatal dysfunction in attention deficit and hyperkinetic disorder. *Archives of Neurology, 46*, 48—52.

Moeschler, J. B., Bennett, F. C. and Cromwell, L. P. (1981). Use of the CT scan in the medical evaluation of the mentally retarded child. *The Journal of Pediatrics, 98*, 63—65.

Morris, R., Blashfield, R., and Satz, P. (1986). Developmental classfication of reading-disabled children. *Journal of Clinical and Experimental Neuropsychology, 8*, 371—392.

Naeser, M. A. and Hayward, R. W. (1978). Lesion localization in aphasia with cranial computed tomography and the Boston Diagnostic Aphasia Examination, *Neurology, 28*, 545—551.

Parkins, R., Roberts, R. J., Reinarz, S. J. and Varney, N. R. (1987, January). CT asymmetries in adult developmental dyslexics. Paper presented at the annual convention of the International Neuropsychological Society, Washington, DC.

Pieniadz, J. M. and Naeser, M. A. (1984). Computed tomographic scan cerebral asymmetries and morphological brain asymmetries. *Archives of Neurology, 41*, 403—409.

Pieniadz, J. M., Naeser, M. A., Koff, E., and Levine, H. L. (1983). CT scan cerebral hemispheric asymmetry measurements in stroke cases with global aphasia: Atypical asymmetries associated with improved recovery. *Cortex, 19*, 371—391.

Rosenberger, P. B. and Hier, D. B. (1980). Cerebral asymmetry and verbal intellectual deficits. *Annals of Neurology, 8*, 300—304.

Rubens, A. B., Mahuwold, M. W., and Hutton, J. T. (1976). Asymmetry of the lateral (sylvian) fissures in man. *Neurology, 26*, 620—624.

Rumsey, J. M., Dorwart, R., Vermess, M., Denckla, M. B., Kruesi, M. J. P., and Rapoport, J. L. (1986). Magnetic resonance imaging of brain anatomy in severe developmental dyslexia. *Arhives of Neurology, 43*, 1045—1046.

Semrud-Clikeman, M., Hynd, G. W., Novey, E. S., and Eliopulos, D. (in press). Dyslexia and brain morphology: Relationships between neuroanatomical variation and neurolinguistic tasks. *Learning and Individual Differences.*

Steinmetz, H., Ebeling, U., Huang, Y., and Kahn, T. (1990). Sulcus topography of the parietal opercular region: An anatomic and MR study. *Brain and Language, 38*, 515—533.

Synek, V., Reuben, J. R., and Duboulay, G. H. (1976). Comparing Evan's index and computerized axial tomography in assessing relationships of ventricular size to brain size. *Neurology, 26*, 231—233.

Taylor, H. G., Fletcher, J. M. (1983). Biological foundations of "specific developmental disorders": Methods, findings, and future directions. *Journal of Clinical Child Psychology, 12*, 46—65.

Teszner, D., Tzavaras, A., Gruner, J., and Hecaen, H. (1972). L'asymetri droite-gauche du planum temporale: A propos de l'etude anatomique de 100 cerveaux. *Revue Neurologique, 126*, 444—449.

Von Economo, C., and Horn, L. (1930). *Zeitschrift fur die gesamte Neurologie und Psyuchiatrie, 130*, 678.

Wada, J. A., Clarke, R., and Hamm, A. (1975). Cerebral hemispheric asymmetry in humans. *Archives of Neurology, 32*, 239—246.

Weinberger, D. R., Luchins, D. J., Morihisa, J., and Wyatt, R. J. (1982). Asymmetrical volumes of the right and left frontal and occipital regions of the human brain. *Neurology, 11*, 97—100.

Witelson, S. F. (1982). Bumps on the brain: Right-left anatomic asymmetry as a key to functional laterialization. In S. Segalowitz (eds.), *Language Functions and Brain Organization* (pp. 117—144). New York: Academic Press.

Witelson, S. F. and Pallie, W. (1973). Left hemisphere specialization for language in the newborn. *Brain, 96*, 641—646.

The Neuropathology of Developmental Dysphasia: Behavioral, Morphological, and Physiological Evidence for a Pervasive Temporal Processing Disorder

PAULA TALLAL, ROBERT L. SAINBURG[1] and TERRY JERNIGAN[2]

[1] *Center for Molecular and Behavioral Neuroscience Rutgers: The State University of New Jersey, Newark, New Jersey;* [2] *Department of Psychiarty, University of California, La Jolla, California*

ABSTRACT: Over the past twenty years, Tallal and colleagues have directed their research toward defining the neuropathological mechanisms responsible for developmental dysphasia. We have hypothesized that higher level auditory processing dysfunction, which has previously been associated with developmental dysphasia, may result from more basic temporal processing deficits which interfere with the resolution of rapidly presented, brief duration stimuli. This temporal processing deficit interferes with adequate perception of specific verbal stimuli which require resolution of brief duration formant transitions, resulting in disordered language development. The temporal processing deficit occurs across multiple sensory modalities, and also affects rapid and sequential motor production skills. Despite relatively normal clinical neuroradiological examinations, *in vivo* morphological analysis, utilizing magnetic resonance imaging techniques for quantitative volumetric measurements of specific brain structures, has identified abnormalities in superior parietal, prefrontal, and temporal cortices, as well as diencephalic and caudate nuclei. Abnormalities in structures which are involved in multimodal processing and sensory motor integration is consistent with the behavioral profile of developmental dysphasia. Two alternative hypotheses regarding the neurophysiological basis of the multimodal temporal processing disorder include: dysfunction in specifc cellular systems which subserve rapid, transient processing; and abnormal gating of sensory relay by intralaminar and reticular thalamic nuclei.

KEYWORDS: developmental dysphasia, dyslexia, temporal processing, MRI, thalamic nuclei, caudate nuclei.

INTRODUCTION

Developmental dysphasia is defined as a specific dysfunction in the development of speech and language expression and/or reception, in the absence of other causal disabilities such as defects of hearing, peripheral speech structures, mental subnormality, personality disorder, brain trauma, or psychoaffective or psychotic disorders (Benton, 1964). The physiological etiology of this disorder is unknown, however recent research has focused on elucidating the neuropsychological, physiological, and possible

Reading and Writing: An Interdisciplinary Journal **3**: 363—377, 1991.
© 1991 *Kluwer Academic Publishers.*

genetic dysfunction underlying this developmental language deficit. The diagnosis is made based on gross behavioral findings, and exclusion of other disorders. Although often termed developmental aphasia, this disorder may differ significantly both in terms of functional deficit and physiological mechanism from the disorder for which the term "aphasia" was coined, traumatic acquired aphasia. Therefore, the disorder will be termed "developmental dysphasia" in this paper, referring to a specific developmental disturbance in language functions, of unknown origin.

This paper will review a series of psychophysical, neuropsychological and anatomical studies which have been directed toward defining the dysfunction of, and elucidating the physiological mechanisms responsible for developmental dysphasia. The research, conducted over the past 20 years by Tallal and colleagues has focused on 4 major areas: analysis of the nonverbal auditory processing deficit association with developmental dysphasia, assessment of the modality specificity of this perceptual deficit and examination of the relationship between the nonverbal processing deficit and verbal dysfunction. Recent work has focused on elucidating the physiological deficit in developmental dysphasia through *in vivo* morphological analysis of brain structures via magnetic resonance imaging (MRI) techniques (Jernigan, Tallal, and Hesselink, 1987; Jernigan, Hesselink, Sowell, and Tallal, in press).

Language processing depends on intact basic sensory reception and processing functions, which culminate in comprehension. These broad steps are necessarily hierarchical, requiring intact signal reception and processing before adequate language comprehension can occur. The basic premise of our research has been the hypothesis that important aspects of acoustic processing are critical for normal speech perception. If acoustic processing is disrupted during development, then this non-verbal processing disorder will interfere with language development.

Behavioral, as well as evoked response audiometry has demonstrated that the peripheral hearing status of children with developmental dysphasia cannot account for their language deficit (Grillon, Couchesne, and Akshoonoff, 1989). In other words, brainstem evoked responses have been found to be relatively normal or, if abnormalities occur, they are insufficient to account for the severity of the language disorder. Despite normal hearing, previous studies have suggested that children with developmental dysphasia have significant "higher level" auditory processing deficits and have focused on two major parameters of auditory perception: auditory sequencing and auditory memory (see Tallal, 1978 for a review). Hirsh (1959) has described these more complex auditory skills as dependent on two more basic abilities: auditory temporal resolution, the perception of two sounds as distinct, and auditory discrimination, the ability to perceive two different sounds as different. Tallal's first set of experiments focused on determining the integrity of these two basic functions in developmentally dysphasic children.

ACOUSTIC PERCEPTION

In order to avoid verbal response requirements, Tallal and Peircy (1973a) developed an operant conditioning paradigm in which subjects were trained to respond to two complex steady state tones of different frequencies presented in rapid succession by pressing one of two response panels. Three basic paradigms were utilized: a same/different paradigm to determine auditory discrimination, a two alternative forced choice paradigm, in which the subjects were required to indicate the order of presentation of the two stimuli by pushing the response panels in the order of stimulus presentation, and a serial memory paradigm, in which the same tones were presented in random order, but in increasingly longer strings of 2, 3, 4, and 5 elements.

In the first set of experiments, twelve 6-9 year old dysphasic children and nine age matched controls were tested. Two 75 msec tones varying in frequency were used. The interstimulus interval (ISI) was varied between 8 and 4062 msec. A criterion of 20/24 correct responses was used. All subjects reached criterion at 428 msec, but the dysphasic's performance rapidly deteriorated with shorter ISI's, with no dysphasic subjects reaching criterion at 305 msec ISI's or shorter. All controls were able to reach criterion at ISI's of 8 msec. A similar pattern of results was demonstrated in the same/different and sequential ordering paradigms. This clearly demonstrated that the sequencing deficit identified in dysphasic children is a secondary sequelea due to the more primary deficit in tone discrimination of rapidly presented stimuli. That is, at rapid rates of presentation, tone stimuli can not be discriminated and therefore, also cannot be sequenced. (i.e., if a subject cannot determine if two stimuli are different, they certainly could not determine the temporal order of those stimuli.)

In the next set of experiments, the role of stimulus duration on auditory perception was examined (Tallal and Piercy, 1973b). The most significant findings were on the serial memory task. Whereas all controls reached criterion on the three element serial memory task at 75 msec stimulus tone durations, only two out of twelve dysphasics reached criterion. However, when stimulus duration was increased to 250 msec, ten out of twelve dysphasics reached criterion on three element patterns. It is significant to note that control performance did not deteriorate significantly as a function of increasing number of elements per sequence, up to five items. However, severe deterioration in the dysphasic subjects' performance was demonstrated at sequence lengths above three elements, even with longer duration stimuli. Thus, it is clear from these results that increasing the duration of the stimulus improves the serial memory performance of dysphasic children, but that serial memory remains impaired in comparison to controls for longer length sequences. Therefore, the time available for acoustic processing is clearly important for sequential memory performance. However, the impairment in serial memory performance may not be entirely attributable to temporal processing deficits, since increasing stimulus duration did not prevent further deterioration in serial memory for tone sequences of greater than three elements. On the other hand, it seems likely that because of the developmental nature of this disorder, the primary temporal processing deficit may cause a form of auditory deprivation. That is, faulty acoustic information processing may deprive the affected children of developmental learning experiences which involve practice with processing clearly differentiated auditory stimuli. The effect of this deprivation may result in, among other things, retarded development of auditory memory skills.

MODALITY SPECIFICITY

The previous experiments clearly indicate an auditory temporal processing deficit in developmentally dysphasic children. The next set of experiments were designed to determine the modality specificity of the temporal processing deficit in developmental dysphasics. In the next series of experiments, the same paradigms described above were presented again; however, in these studies, visual presentation of 2 light stimuli (2 shades of green) replaced the auditory tones (Tallal and Peircy, 1973b). The same subjects were tested again with visual stimuli. No significant group differences were found, which indicated that the temporal processing deficit was specific to the auditory modality. However, these results do not rule out the possibility of a general cross modality temporal processing disorder, in which the specific stimulus quality and temporal constraints vary according to modality. The use of shading differences was chosen because a subtle difference in light frequency appeared at least physically analogous to sound frequency differences. However, the neural mechanisms responsible for the discrimination of sound frequency differences may be more analogous to other types of visual discrimination such as orientation or form discrimination. Therefore this study did provide evidence against cross modality effects of the temporal processing deficit, but in itself was inconclusive.

In a later set of experiments (Tallal, Stark, Kallman, and Mellits, 1981), the paradigm was modified to examine modality specificity of temporal processing across a larger age span. In these experiments, three types of visual stimuli were used: two shades of green, two nonsense letter-like characters (ε and ϕ), and two letters (E and K). In these experiments, shorter ISI's resulted in equally impaired performance on both auditory and visual tasks for dysphasics ranging in age from 5 to 6 yrs. However, performance on auditory tasks among the 7 and 8 year olds was two times worse than performance on visual tasks. Therefore, the temporal processing deficit appeared to be general, across modalities in the younger age group, but was selective to the auditory modality in the older group. One explanation for this discrepancy may be that the cross sectional sample may have been skewed according to age group, with greater diversity in the degree and scope of impairment in the younger group. Only the most seriously impaired children may continue to be specifically language impaired at the older ages and thus may represent a more homogeneous disorder. On the other hand, differential temporal parameters may govern the processing of sequentially presented visual or auditory stimuli during the course of normal development. In other words, at the younger ages the auditory and visual systems may be functioning under similar temporal constraints, while the visual system may function under different time constraints than the auditory system in the older group. The presentation parameters used for the perception paradigm may not be sensitive enough to pick up significant errors on visual tasks in the older group.

In summary, it is clear that the younger age group demonstrated a lack of modality specificity in their temporal processing disorder. However, the ability of the paradigm to resolve visual temporal processing deficits in older children may be poor due to age dependent changes in the visual system, or due to group variance differences across ages.

In an additional set of experiments, a battery of clinical neurological and neuropsychological tests were given to dysphasic children revealing significant deficits in discrimination of simultaneously presented tactile stimuli, and deficits in producing rapid alternating and sequential movements (Katz, Tallal and Curtiss, submitted; Tallal, Stark, and Mellits, 1985a; Johnson, Stark, Mellits, and Tallal, 1981). Based on these findings, it appears that the perceptual deficit associated with developmental dysphasia may affect multiple modalities. It is unclear if the dysfunction in producing rapid motor behaviors is due to primary efferent system deficits, or whether these effects are secondary to deficits in somatosensory processing. Although the majority of data indicates a temporal processing deficit, dysphasic children demonstrated poor tactile discrimination to simultaneously presented stimuli. This may be representative of a dysfunction in temporal resolution (i.e., ISI = 0), or spatial resolution. Whether the deficit involves primarily temporal processing or spatial processing may vary depending on the modality. Indeed, spatial resolution is a more salient feature of tactile perception than auditory perception. More specific studies of the somatosensory involvement in developmental dysphasia is required to answer this question. It is however, physiologically consistent for a temporal and spatial resolution deficit to exist concurrently, since both spatial and temporal gating mechanisms probably involve similar lateral and recurrent inhibition mechanisms.

One mechanim which may be hypothesized to account for the temporal processing deficits seen in developmental dysphasics is a temporal gating mechanism involving "edge sharpening" of stimuli. Edge sharpening, as used here, refers to the clarification of receptive field edges by lateral inhibition mechanisms, thereby providing a perceptual "window" for stimulus resolution. Such lateral inhibition mechanisms have been described for visual, tactile, and auditory systems (Berne and Levy, 1988). Temporal edge sharpening may involve recurrent feedback mechanisms which function to gate the frequency of incoming sensory impulses, and therefore provide, perceptually, a temporal discrimination window. Clearly a common dysfunction in "edge sharpening" functions may be occurring across modalities in developmental dysphasics.

A second hypothesis has been raised by Livingstone, who suggested that the parallel magnocellular and parvocellular systems identified in the visual system may have counterparts in other modalities (Livingstone and Galaburda, 1990). These two pathways remain relatively segregated throughout the visual system. At the level of the retinal ganglion cells through the lateral geniculate, the response properties of the two systems vary significantly (Perry, Oehler, and Cowey, 1984). The magnocellular system receives input mostly from peripheral retinal photoreceptors, has low spatial resolution, is not color coded, has little contrast sensitivity, and responds best to high frequency stimuli. On the other hand, the parvocellular system receives mostly from central retina, has high spatial resolution, is color coded, is highly contrast sensitive, and responds best to low frequency stimuli (Perry and Shapely, 1986; Kaplan and Shapley, 1982). The magnocellular system appears designed to respond best to rapid, transient or moving stimuli presented in peripheral fields, while the parvocellular system responds best to detailed, static stimuli presented foveally. Livingstone proposed that similar functionally segregated parallel subsystems could exist in a variety of sensory systems. Selective impairment in the subsystems subserving fast transient responses may underlie the temporal processing deficit in developmental dysphasia. In opposition to this hypothesis, the errors in visual discrimination presented above, while temporally dependent, occurred in response to color differences, as well as detailed form differences in black and white stimuli, which were regarded foveally. The role of the magnocellular system in processing these stimuli would be expected to be minimal. However, it is possible that activation of the magnocellular system during rapid transient stimulation is necessary for adequate parvocellular processing. A more detailed analysis of the visual processing deficits which occur across stimuli selected specifically to represent each of these two visual subsystems would provide a better understanding of the possible neural dysfunction underlying developmental dysphasia.

VERBAL PERCEPTION

The previously described psychoacoustic work supported the hypothesis that a temporal processing deficit is primary to developmental dysphasia, and may be prerequisite to the speech and language dysfunction. Based on an understanding of how phonemes transmit information about speech, various predictions were made. Specific elements of the acoustic signal within a phoneme are essential for perceptual discrimination. For example, steady-state vowels transmit the same acoustic information throughout their spectra. However, stop consonant-vowel syllables have a transitional period between the release of the consonant and the initiation of the vowel during which the frequencies change very rapidly in time. Information carried within these brief formant transitions is critical for syllable discrimination. We predicted that dysphasic children would be unimpaired in discriminating between speech sounds which are characterized by steady-state acoustic spectra, such as vowels. On the other hand, they would be significantly impaired in discriminating speech sounds such as stop consonant-vowel syllables, which incorporate very rapidly changing formant transitions. Experimental results were consistent with these predictions (Tallal and Peircy, 1974, 1975). The critical stimulus parameter interfering with successful performance on discrimination tasks proved to be the rate of temporal change, not whether the stimulus was verbal or nonverbal.

A subsequent experiment was carried out to determine if the poor performance found on tests with stop consonant-vowel syllables was due to impaired ability to process transitional elements of auditory information or simply due to the short duration of the stimulus period (Tallal and Peircy, 1975). In this experiment the previous paradigms were carried out with computer generated speech stimuli that were modified to change their temporal components. Vowel-vowel syllables were constructed to include approximately 50 msec steady state durations, while stop consonant-vowel syllables were constructed with synthetically extended formant transitions. Results demonstrated that the dysphasics' performance on tests using steady-state vowel sounds, but of brief duration, was significantly impaired. Conversely, extending the formant transition within stop consonant-vowel syllables resulted in significantly improved performance. Thus, the clear conclusion of these studies was that a highly specific auditory temporal deficit is sufficient to interfere with the perception of brief duration acoustic information essential for normal speech discrimination, regardless of whether or not stimuli are transitional or steady-state. Subsequent studies demonstrated a highly significant relation between the degree of temporal processing deficit and the extent of receptive language impairment in dysphasic children (Tallal, Stark, and Mellits, 1985b).

There may also be a striking convergence of data between dysphasic and dyslexic children. Longitudinal studies have demonstrated that the vast majority of developmental dysphasic children have inordinate difficulty learning to read (see Tallal, Curtiss, and Kaplan, 1988 for a review). A broad body of research now suggests that phonological awareness and coding deficits may be at the heart of developmental reading disorders

(Liberman, 1988). But, what is the physiological basis of disorders in phonological awareness and coding? Struck by the considerable overlap between developmental dysphasia and dyslexia, Tallal and colleagues carried out experiments with two groups of dyslexic children. One group had depressed scores not only on standardized reading tests, but on measures of oral language as well. The other group was equally impaired in reading, but was within normal limits on tests of oral language. The phonological coding, as well as temporal processing abilities of these two groups of dyslexics were assessed and compared to that of dysphasic children. The results were clear. The dyslexic children with concomitant oral language disabilities had significant deficits in both phonological coding (reading nonsense words) and non-verbal temporal processing. Furthermore, these deficits were highly correlated with each other in these dyslexics ($r = 0.81$). Interestingly, the dyslexics with normal oral language scores had neither phonological coding or temporal processing deficits. Thus, deficits in basic temporal processing may interfere with phoneme analysis leading to initial speech perception and/or language deficits, and subsequent deficits in phonological awareness and reading development (Tallal, 1980; Tallal and Stark, 1982; Stark and Tallal *et al.*, 1988). It is particularly relevant to note that genetic studies have found that decoding deficits in reading nonsense words may be among the best phenotype markers for developmental dyslexia (see Olson, Gillis, Rack, and DeFries, in press; Stevenson, in press).

Our studies suggest that the physiological basis of phoneme awareness deficits in dyslexia may be basic temporal integration and serial memory deficits, and that it may be these deficits which are transmitted genetically. A recent study completed in Tallal's laboratory lends direct support to this hypothesis. Language/reading impaired (L/RI)[1] children with other affected first degree relatives were compared to matched L/RI children without other affected family members. Few behavioral differences in phenotype emerged. However, a significant group difference was found on a battery of nonverbal auditory attention and temporal processsing tests, with L/RI children with a positive family history for language and/or learning disability performing significantly more poorly than those without a positive family history (Tallal, Townsend, Curtiss, and Wulfeck, in press). Taken together, these data suggest that there may be a continuum between developmental language disorders and the types of reading disorders which are characterized by deficits in phonological awareness. The genetic basis for this continua may be in a physiological deficit which slows the rate of basic sensory information processing in the nervous system. The search for an anatomical/morphological substrate for such a deficit was investigated in the following series of studies.

[1] L/RI refers to children selected at age 4 as developmental dysphasics and followed longitudinally to age 8, at which time they were both language and reading impaired.

CEREBRAL MORPHOLOGY

A series of studies of cerebral morphology, utilizing magnetic resonance imaging (MRI) to calculate volumetric data, was undertaken recently by Jernigan and Tallal (Jernigan, Tallal, and Hesselink, 1987; Jernigan, Hesselink, Sowell, and Tallal, in press). Volumetric measurements of cerebral grey matter, both cortical and subcortical was obtained for twenty language impaired and twelve control subjects in the age range of 8 to 10 years. The sample was drawn from a larger sample of ninety five specifically language impaired children and sixty age, nonverbal I.Q., race, and SES matched controls who were identified at 4 years old and studied longitudinally until age 8. The method of utilizing magnetic resonance imaging techniques for *in vivo* quantitative volumetric analysis of brain morphology presents a powerful, and non-invasive technique for exploring the anatomical and physiological basis of chronic, non life-threatening nervous system disorders such as developmental dysphasia. Therefore, the methods will be explained here in some depth (see Jernigan *et al.*, in press, for a more detailed discussion).

The following techniques were utilized to define and quantify brain structure volumes from MRI data. To facilitate and standardize the determination of structure edges, the method involved a semi-automated classification of each voxel within a brain section on the basis of its signal characteristics on two spatially registered MR images of that section. These classifications corresponded to major tissue types: grey matter, white matter, cerebral spinal fluid (CSF), and tissue abnormalities. The full series of axial brain sections was analyzed, beginning at the bottom of the cerebellar hemispheres and extending through the vertex.

Specific brain structures were then defined. Subcortical structures were identified by visually identifying groups of pixels classified as grey matter which were located within caudate nuclei, lenticular nuclei, and diencephalic grey matter structures (including mammillary bodies, hypothalamic grey, septal nuclei, and thalamus). Cerebral regions were defined relative to the centromedial structural midline and two consistently identifiable points: the most anterior point on the genu, and the most posterior point on the splenium of the corpus callosum. By calculating rotation angles using these landmarks, it was possible to perform a three dimensional rotation of the images, thus correcting each individual's image data for rotation out of the optimal imaging plane. Regions could then be constructed which resulted in highly consistent placement of regional boundaries relative to gross anatomical landmarks.

Six cerebral zones were identified relative to these planes: IA_1, IA_2, IP_1, IP_2, SA, SP. The first letter of the region describes its position relative to the axial dividing plane (inferior or superior), and the second to the coronal plane (anterior or posterior). Thus, IA is inferior to the axial and anterior to the coronal plane. This division resulted in the inclusion of all posterior perisylvian cortical structures in the IP zones, however the occipital lobe was also included in this zone. In addition, the IA zone included both anterior temporal and frontal cortical structures. In order to separate IA and IP into more anatomically distinct regions, two additional coronal dividing planes were added which subdivided the region inferior to the axial plane. The resulting six cerebral regions are defined in the table below and shown in figure 1.

Group comparisons were made on: cerebral asymmetry of the volumes of each of the six regions, and absolute hemispheric volumes of cerebral and subcortical structures. Asymmetry was expressed as a ratio of the total voxel quantity of the left hemisphere region to the total voxel quantity of the homologous right hemisphere region.

Results revealed generally unremarkable findings on routine clinical neuroradiological examination. However, quantitative volumetric analysis revealed significant morphological differences in dysphasic children vs.

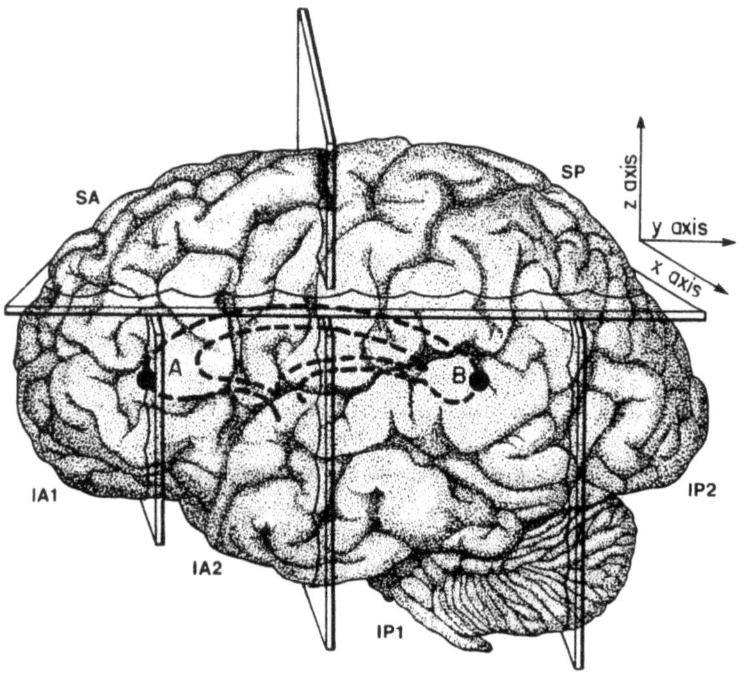

Fig. 1: Figure 1 shows the six brain regions used for morphometric analysis to compare MR images from language impaired and control children. SA = Superior Anterior; SP = Superior Posterior; IA_1 = Inferior Anterior 1; IA_2 = Inferior Anterior 2; IP_1 = Inferior Posterior 1; IP_2 = Inferior Posterior 2

Table 1. Summary of cortical structures within each cerebral region

Inferior Anterior 1 (IA_1):	
	Prefrontal cortex inferior to a plane above the frontal operculum, including orbitofrontal, dorsolateral and mesial frontal lobe.
Inferior Anterior 2 (IA_2):	
	The temporal poles, uncus, and some amygdala.
	Anterior perforated substance and adjacent orbitofrontal cortex.
	Anterior insular cortex and frontal operculum.
Inferior Posterior 1 (IP_1):	
	Most of temporal cortex, including all mesial temporal lobe structures posterior to the amygdala (only the temporal pole is included in IA2).
	Peri-sylvian parietal cortex and parietal operculum.
Inferior Posterior 2 (IP_2):	
	Most of the occipital lobe (only a small portion of the superior occipital cortex was included in SP).
	A small part of the most posterior gyri of the temporal lobe on the lateral cortical surface.
Superior Anterior (SA):	
	Superior parts of the dorsolateral and mesial frontal lobes (above the frontal operculum).
Superior Posterior (SP):	
	Superior parietal lobe above the parietal operculum.
	A small portion of the most superior occupital lobe.

Note: From Jernigan et al., in press

controls. Results indicated significantly different asymmetries in dysphasics vs. controls for both IA_1 and SP regions.

In IA_1, or prefrontal cortex, controls demonstrated symmetry between the two hemispheres, while dysphasics demonstrated a smaller volume in the left than in the right hemisphere. In SP, the superior parietal and parieto-occipital regions, controls showed larger right than left volumes, while dysphasics showed the opposite pattern (left larger than right). In terms of comparisons of absolute volumes, the IP_1 or posterior peri-sylvian region (the region which has been most clearly associated with receptive language function), was significantly reduced bilaterally in dysphasics. In addition, subcortical volumes in the right diencephalon and caudate were also significantly reduced in dysphasics compared to controls. Ratios of tissue type: grey matter, white matter, and CSF were similar for dysphasics and controls.

It is clear from this work that although routine clinical neuroradiological examinations revealed no significant structural defects in developmentally dysphasic children, abnormalities in brain morphology were significant when measured quantitatively. There is evidence of bilateral reduction in the perisylvian volume, the brain region which has been most clearly related to functional receptive language deficits. Significant morphological abnormalities were also demonstrated in posterior parietal and prefrontal cortices, as well as diencephalic and caudate nuclei. These structures represent areas of multimodality sensory processing and sensory motor integration. Thus, the behavioral results from Tallal's laboratory, revealing a significant multimodal temporal processing deficit, are consistent with morphological abnormalities in these structures.

Preliminary analysis aimed at directly linking the verbal and temporal perceptual deficits of L/RI children with the morphological differences found on MRI have proved promising. Significant correlations are found between degree of volumetric reduction in the left IP_1 region and a reduction in verbal IQ score. Similarly, significant correlations have emerged between auditory sequential memory performance and hemispheric asymmetry ratio differences in the IA_1 and SP regions. More detailed analysis are currently in progress to reveal the precise pattern of relationship between functional and structural patterns in L/RI children.

SUMMARY

Major results from this line of research demonstrate the involvement of a significant deficit in temporal analysis of auditory information, which predicts both the pattern of speech perception and production deficits, as well as the degree of receptive language deficit in developmental dysphasia. In addition, the evidence implicates cross modality gating mechanisms, possibly involving a deficit in temporal and spatial "edge sharpening" functions. The morphological findings from MRI studies implicate cortical as well as subcortical structures. It is possible to speculate that during neurogenesis, a primary subcortical structure fails to develop normally, resulting in the spectrum of morphological deficits seen in L/RI children. Given the subcortical involvement demonstrated on volumetric analysis together with the behavioral deficits in temporal processing and motor control which have been shown to characterize these children, we hypothesize that thalamic gating mechanisms may be involved. The results of evoked potential studies suggest that the deficit may involve normal input to brainstem and thalamus, but abnormal thalamic or post-thalamic processing. The widespread cortical morphological involvement, including the temporal lobes bilaterally, as well as parietal and frontal association cortices, supports the involvement of subcortical structures which provide widespread input to cortex, as well as reciprocal innervation of nonprimary cortices. In addition, based on the MRI data, the primary affected structure would also be expected to provide heavy innervation of caudate nucleus, since this structure is also significantly reduced in volume in the brains of L/RI children.

Nuclei which receive input from all modalities as well as from widespread cortical regions include the nonspecific nuclei of the thalamus. The intralaminar nuclei have reciprocal innervations with caudate nucleus, widespread nonprimary cortical sites, and thalamic reticular nuclei (Macchi and Bentivoglio, 1986). The reticular nuclei have been shown to provide powerful inhibitory input to specific thalamic nuclei (Macchi and Bentivoglio, 1986). Since reticular nuclei receive input from the same specific thalamic sites to which they project, these nuclei provide a possible mechanism for recurrent feedback mechanisms.

A possible thalamic mechanism involved in temporal gating of sensory information in the temporal range shown to be disordered in dysphasic children (20 hz to 5 hz) may involve, in part, intrathalamic circuits which involve input from specific "relay" nuclei, and which provide feedback to the same nuclei. The intralaminar and reticular nuclei provide a possible anatomical substrate for such an interaction. In addition, the mechanism would be expected to be modulated by association cortical areas, where judgements regarding priority and relevance of information would be expected to be made. Again, the anatomical substrate is relevant. The nonspecific nuclei input to specific "relay" cells, may provide a filtering function by modulating the excitability of these cells following phasic activation. This could be achieved through modulation of specific potassium conductances, such as IA or calcium dependent conductances which would result in altered after-hyperpolarization durations (see Strong and Kaczmarek, 1987, for a detailed discussion of these potassium conductances). Based on behavioral work, implicating a multiple modality temporal gating mechanism, and morphological work implicating nonprimary cortical, diencephalic and striatal involvement, it may be hypothesized that nonspecific thalamic nuclei are involved in the primary pathology of developmental dysphasia. In support of such a hypothesis, there is a growing body of evidence that damage to thalamic structures results in acquired aphasic disorders in some adult patients (Jones, 1982; Luria, 1977; Moher, Watter, and Duncan, 1975). Similarly, Ojemann described language production and verbal memory deficits as a result of nongeniculate thalamic lesions and in response to thalamic electrical stimulation (Ojemann, 1984).

The proposed mechanism is a speculative integration of these behavioral and morphological findings into a single primary structural pathology. An alternative hypothesis is that single developmental events, such as the presence of abnormal cell adhesion proteins, may result in a wide spectrum of structural abnormalities which are functionally and anatomically unrelated, or which represent a dysfunction in similar cellular systems across multiple modalities, such as the magnocellular components of the visual system. However, in support of a mechanism which functionally integrates the morphological data, preliminary results have indicated a significant correlation between extent of morphological involvement and the severity of the language deficit. As such, the studies described in this paper provide a solid foundation upon which to base further research into the specific neurophysiological basis of the temporal modulation mechanism which appears to be primary in the neuropathology of specific developmental language and reading disorders.

REFERENCES

Benton, A. L. (1964). Developmental aphasia and brain damage. *Cortex, 1*, 40—52.

Berne, R., and Levy, M. (1988). *Physiology* (2nd ed.). Washington, D.C.: The C. V. Mosby Co. (pp. 106—111, 140, 176).

Grillon, C., Courchesne, E., and Akshoonoff, N. (1989). Brainstem and middle latency auditory evoked potentials in autism and developmental language disorder. *Journal of Autism and Developmental Disorders, 19*(2), 255—69.

Hirsh, I. J. (1959). Auditory perception of temporal order. *Journal of the Acoustic Society of America, 3*, 157—78.

Jernigan, T., Hesselink J., Sowell, E., and Tallal, P. (in press). Cerebral morphology on MRI in language-learnıng children. *Archives of Neurology.*

Jernigan, T., Tallal, P., and Hesselink, J. (1987). Cerebral morphology on magnetic resonance imaging in developmental dysphasia. *Society of Neuroscience Abstracts, 13*(1), 651.

Johnson, R., Stark, R., Mellits, E., and Tallal, P. (1981). Neurological status of language impaired and normal children. *Annals of Neurology, 10*, 159—163.

Jones, S. (1982). The thalamus and aphasia, including transcortical aphasia: a review. *Journal of Communication Disorders, 15*(1), 31—44.

Kaplan, E., and Shapely, R. (1982). X and Y cells in the lateral geniculate of macaque monkeys. *Journal of Phsıology (London), 330*, 125—146.

Katz, W. F., Tallal, P., and Curtiss, D. S. (Submitted). Rapid autmomatized naming and gestures by normal and language impaired children.

Liberman, I. Y. (1988). Phonology and beginning reading revisisted. In Von Euler, Lundberg, and Lennerstrand (eds.). *Braın and Reading* (pp. 112—143) London: Mac Millan Press.

Livingstone, M. and Galaburda, A. (1990). Physiological evidence for a magnocellular defect in development dyslexia. Paper presented at the National Dyslexia Research Foundation Conference: The exceptional Brain, Barcelona, Spain.

Luria, A. R. (1977). On quasi-aphasic disturbances in lesions of deep structures of the brain. *Brain and Language, 4*(3), 432—459.

Macchi, G., and Bentivoglio, M. (1986). The thalamic intralaminar nuclei and the cerebral cortex. In E. Jones and A. Peters (eds.), Cerebral Cortex (pp. 335—401). New York: Plenum Press.

Moher, J., Watter, W., and Duncan, G. (1975). Thalamic hemorrhage and aphasia. *Braın and Language, 2*, 3—17.

Ojemann, G. A. (1984). Common cortical and thalamic mechanisms for language and motor functions. *American Journal of Physiological, 15* 901—903.

Olson, R. K., Gillis, J. J., Rack, J. P., DeFries, J. C., and Fulker, D. W. (in press). Confirmatory factor analysis of word recognition and process measures in the Colorado Reading Project. *Reading and Writing: An Interdisciplinary Journal.*

Perry, V., Oehler, R., and Cowey, A. (1984). Retinal ganglion cells that project to the dorsal lateral geniculate nucleus in the macaque monkey. *Neuroscience, 12,* 1101–1122.

Perry, V., and Shapley, R. (1986). Cat and monkey retinal ganglion cells and their functional roles. *Trends in Neurosciences, 9,* 1–9.

Stark, R. E., and Tallal, P. (1988). *Language, Speech, and Reading Disorders in Children: Neurobiological Studies.* San Diego: College Hall Press.

Stevenson, J. (in press). Which aspects of processing text mediate genetic effects? *Reading and Writing: An Interdiciplinary Journal.*

Strong, J., and Kaczmarek, L. (1987). Potassium currents that regulate action potentials and repetitive firing. In L. Kaczmarek and I. Levitan (eds.), *Neuromodulation* (pp. 119–134). New York: Oxford University Press.

Tallal, P. (1978). An experimental investigation of the role of auditory temporal processing in normal and disordered language development. In A. Caramazza and E. Zurif (eds.), *Language Acquisition and Language Breakdown: Parallels and Divergences* (pp. 25–61). Baltimore, MD: The John Hopkins University Press.

Tallal, P. (1980). Auditory temporal perception, phonics and reading disabilities in children. *Brain and Language, 9,* 182–198.

Tallal, P., Curtiss, S., and Kaplan, R. (1988). The San Diego longitudinal study: Evaluating the outcomes of preschool impairment in language development. In S. E. Gerber and G. T. Mencher (eds.), *Interntional perspectives on communication disorders* (pp. 86–126). Washington, DC: Gallaudet University Press.

Tallal, P., and Peircy, M. (1973a). Defects of non-verbal auditory perception in children with developmental aphasia. *Nature, 241,* 468–469.

Tallal, P., and Peircy, M. (1973b). Developmental aphasia: impaired rate of non-verbal processing as a function of sensory modality. *Neuropsychologia, 11,* 389–398.

Tallal, P., and Peircy, M. (1974). Developmental aphasia: Rate of auditory processing and selective impairment of consonant perception. *Neuropsychologia, 12,* 83–93.

Tallal, P., and Peircy, M. (1975). Developmental Aphasia: The perception of brief vowels and extended stop consonants. *Neurosychologia, 13,* 69–74.

Tallal, P., and Stark, R. (1982). Perceptual/motor profiles of reading impaired children with or without concomitant oral language deficits. *Annuals of Dyslexia, 32,* 163–176.

Tallal, P., Stark, R., Kallman, C., and Mellits, E. (1981). A reexamination of some non-verbal perceptual abilities of language impaired and normal children as a function of age and sensory modality. *Journal of Speech and Hearing Research, 24,* 351–357.

Tallal, P., Stark, R., and Mellits, E. (1985a). Identification of language impaired children on the basis of rapid perception and production skills. *Brain and Language, 25,* 314–322.

Tallal, P., Stark, R., and Mellits, E. (1985b). The relationship between auditory analysis and receptive language development: Evidence from studies of developmental language disorder. *Neuropsychologia, 23,* 527–534.

Tallal, P., Townsend, J., Curtiss, S., and Wulfeck, B. (in press). Phenotypic profiles of language impaired children based on genetic/family history. *Brain and Language.*

Investigation of Abnormal Left Temporal Functioning in Dyslexia Through rCBF, Auditory Evoked Potentials, and Positron Emisson Tomography

FRANK WOOD,[1] LYNN FLOWERS[1], MONTE BUCHSBAUM[2] and PAULA TALLAL[3]

[1] *Bowman Gray School of Medicine Winston-Salem, NC;* [2] *Brain Imaging Center University of California, Irvine;* [3] *Center for Molecular and Behavioral Neuroscience, Rutgers, Newark, NJ*

ABSTRACT: The proposed left hemisphere dysfunction in dyslexia was investigated in a review of four studies using regional cerebral blood flow (rCBF; N = 152) and combined auditory evoked responses (AERs) with positron emission tomography (PET) (N = 20). In contrast to the positive relation that was found between temporal rCBF and orthographic task accuracy, an inverse correlation was found phonemic in normals between task accuracy and left temporal rCBF activation, near Heschl's gyrus. Dyslexics, by contrast, showed a positive correlation between Heschl's gyrus activation (by PET and rCBF) and phonemic processing accuracy. The AER's at C3 for an early positive component (P1) showed that these relationships were true both on hit trials and correct rejection trials, indicating that the perceptual rather than motoric or selective attention aspects of the task were being measured. Methodological issues were emphasized, including the difficulty of interpreting mean differences in brain activity at a given site without considering the separate multivariate structures that might exist in the two populations.

KEYWORDS: Dyslexia, reading disability, neuroimaging, auditory evoked responses, regional cerebral blood flow, positron emission tomography, left temporal dysfunction.

INTRODUCTION

Increasingly, studies of the abnormality in developmental dyslexia have implicated fundamental language mechanisms on the behavioral side (Vellutino, 1979; Pennington, et al., 1987; Felton and Wood, 1989; Felton, Naylor, Wood, 1990) and a left hemisphere, particularly left frontotemporal, substrate on the neuroanatomical side (Galaburda, et al., 1985; Kaufman and Galaburda, 1989). While these investigations are somewhat compelling in their emphasis on certain core mechanisms of phonological and verbal information processing deficit, the functional neuroanatomical substrate has been as yet less accurately delimited and specified. If the mechanisms of disorder could be characterized with the same precision in the functional neuroanatomical domain as they have been characterized in the behavioral domain, then the stage would be set

Reading and Writing: An Interdisciplinary Journal 3: 379—393, 1991.
© 1991 *Kluwer Academic Publishers.*

for fundamental advance in the neuropsychology of abnormal brain function in general as well as in dyslexia particularly.

In previous reviews (Wood, 1983; Wood and Felton, 1983; Wood, 1990), we have considered general issues in functional neuroimaging of normal and pathological brain behavior relations in humans. In this paper, we apply some of these general principles to the above problem of left temporal functional abnormality in dyslexia — illustrating the application by reference to our series of functional neuroimaging studies of dyslexics and normal controls. For a related treatment of the methodological issues relating to temporal lobe anatomical differences, see Galaburda and Steinmetz (1991).

The possibility of anomalous left hemisphere functioning in dyslexia arises both from microneural and macroneural investigations.

1. On the microneural side are the post-mortem cytoarchitectural differences in dyslexic brains, particularly in left peri-Sylvian areas (Galaburda et al., 1985; Kaufman and Galaburda, 1989; Duane, 1989). These implicate early, embryonic cell migration forming the upper cortical layers. Of special note is the fact that these relatively small changes, occurring at this critical time when connectivities are being established, could well cause larger — and functionally significant — alterations of organized neural functioning.

2. Macroneural changes include the absence — in reading disabled subjects — of the normal left-greater-than-right asymmetry in the posterior temporal planum (Tp) in autopsy material (Galaburda et al., 1985; Kaufman and Galaburda, 1989) and in magnetic resonance imaging (Larsen, Hoien, Lundberg and Odegaard, 1990). This symmetry generally involves abnormally larger right temporal plana, not smaller left temporal plana, in dyslexics. There are existence proofs in animals that abnormal bilateral enlargements of remote cortical areas can arise from early unilateral lesions, as in Goldman (1978) and Goldman-Rakic and Rakic (1984). It is, therefore, at least possible — though completely unproven — that symmetrical temporal plana could also be a consequence (or "symptom") of an early unilateral lesion, perhaps left peri-Sylvian in locus.

There is also physiological evidence for language related functional organization of the left hemisphere. The intraoperative brain electrical stimulation studies of seizure patients by Ojemann (1983) are particularly useful: they employ momentary, localized electrical disruptions of cortical functioning in awake humans — making the *functional* equivalent of temporary cortical lesions and observing their impact on language performance. These studies identify sites whose temporary lesioning abolishes core language skills such as naming, orofacial sequencing, and phonetic discrimination. In persons with normal verbal intelligence, these sites are generally distributed closely along both banks of the left Sylvian fissure (Ojemann, 1983; Ojemann and Whitaker, 1978). Males with verbal IQ's below 90, however, showed a posterior displacement of naming-related sites, away from the superior temporal gyrus and toward the angular gyrus.

Rasmussen and Milner (1977) have similarly related early left temporal-Wernicke's area lesions to a posterior redistribution of some language functions. The implication is once again that an early left temporal lesion may initiate functional reorganization — in this case within the hemisphere.

The above studies imply altered functional organization in dyslexia — an implication well suited to the functional neuroimaging techniques, because of their capability for simultaneous measurement of activation at many cortical (and, with PET, subcortical) locations during actual language or reading-related performance. Indeed, altered functional organization can, by definition, only be studied with simultaneous measurement of many local brain areas no single measurements of a particular site can ever disclose functions that may have been reorganized or displaced from that site.

Within the set of functional neuroimaging techniques, the various methods each have their strengths and weaknesses. The 133-Xenon regional cerebral blood flow (rCBF) method is particularly well-suited for monitoring the macro-neural correlates of language activation: the temporal resolution permits a task lasting only a few minutes; the relative safety and low cost allow the use of large normal reference groups and multiple conditions (Wood, 1980 and 1983); and resolution of the gray versus white matter flow exceeds that of other methods. Positron emission tomography (PET) obviously allows much finer spatial resolution, including subcortical, but sacrifices temporal resolution when glucose utilization is measured, since the uptake period (and therefore the task performance) is about 40 minutes long. At the other extreme, event-related potentials (ERP's) achieve maximal temporal resolution, in milliseconds, but at the cost of spatial resolution both absolutely (because of the relatively small number of electrodes) and relatively (because of the difficulty of source localization of scalp measured potentials). Ideally, then, the techniques would be jointly employed, so that the weaknesses of one would be compensated by the strengths of another.

Experiment 1

Correlation of task accuracy with regional cerebral blood flow measured during task performance.

In this experiment, reported elsewhere in detail (Flowers, Wood, Naylor, 1991, Study 1), left temporal activation was examined in a group of normals performing an auditory orthographic analysis task. We used an orthographic analysis task to activate a reading-relevant neural process during the measurement of regional blood flow. Sixty-nine normal right handed subjects (39 male and 30 female) listened to common concrete nouns — one every 2.5 seconds — and indicated with a bilateral finger lift response whether the word was exactly four letters long: a random half of the words met this target criterion. Hits and False Alarms were used to calculate an unbiased accuracy score, d-prime (Green and Swets, 1966).

Regional cerebral blood flow (rCBF) was measured by the 133-Xenon inhalation method. Sixteen NaI (T1)-crystal scintillation collimators, eight per hemisphere held in place by a helmet, collected gamma emissions in five second bins. Probe locations were chosen to reflect sensory, motor, attentional, and language processing areas. After one minute of Xenon inhalation, the tracer clearance rate for each probe was measured over the next ten minutes yielding a value representing a conservative estimate of gray matter activation (after the method of Prohovnik et al., 1985). This Initial Slope Index (ISI) was the dependent measure.

Our prediction of left temporal activation from this task was tested by a correlation between left temporal flow (expressed as a ratio to hemispheric mean) and task accuracy (measured as d-prime). The result was clear: of all sites, only left temporal flow was significantly correlated with task accuracy. The correlation was positive, so that subjects performing with greater accuracy showed greater left temporal flow (relative to the mean hemispheric flow). This finding was statistically independent of and unrelated to gender, age, education, and state anxiety (Spielberger, et al., 1983).

Several methodological issues are raised by this experiment, and they have direct relevance for dyslexia studies. First, this result suggests the importance of left temporal lobe activity in the normal execution of the task, but it certainly does not specify what aspect of the task was responsible for the correlation with left temporal flow. Was it the auditory processing of the words themselves, or the orthographic analysis, that was correlated with left temporal flow?

The question cannot even be considered until a second, major issue is faced: Should we expect positive or negative correlations with task accuracy? The question is reviewed at length in Wood (1983; 1990), in which examples of both types of correlations are considered. In general, it appears that negative correlations imply a task that is usually well automatized in normal individuals, so that those finding it difficult (and doing it correspondingly poorly) are actually expending greater effort, including neural effort. In such tasks, practice has not only made perfect but has also made relatively effortless. On the other hand, tasks requiring either the recruitment of novel, less well-practiced, strategies or the integration of separate items of information in novel ways, might well be best performed by those who expend the most effort at such recruitment or integration. In that case, more is better.

In that context, then, we might expect that it is the more novel aspects of the task — involving word retrieval, the translation of familiar, whole words to orthographic code, letter counting, and memory — that are the ones positively correlating with left temporal flow. In contrast, the actual auditory comprehension of the phonemes and words themselves, might actually be negatively correlated with temporal flow. In this case, however, the task is designed to minimize variance from that source by making the words familiar and easy to understand. Little impact of individual differences at the more automatized perceptual level is expected, therefore; still less could it be measured.

Furthermore, the study presents distinctive issues in its use of a correlational strategy to assess localized functioning. Often, studies such as this use a resting baseline, or another control task performance, as conditions during which flow should also be measured and then compared to flow engendered during the experimental task in question. Differences in flow from baseline to experimental task, or from control task to experimental task, are then assigned, by classical subtraction logic to these differences in task or state. Such designs can isolate more particular features of task performance than are isolated by the task accuracy correlation (since a variety of influences might be affecting task accuracy). However, the correlational design calls attention to the particular feature of most interest in dyslexia studies — the prospect of individual differences in temporal lobe activation "ability." This logic invites a second experiment, involving measured differences in ability — here childhood reading — to see if indeed these ability differences are directly related to temporal lobe flow.

Experiment 2

Reorganization of Left Temporo-Parietal Flow During Orthographic Analysis in Adults with a History of Childhood Dyslexia.

This experiment (reported as Studies 2 and 3 in Flowers, Wood, and Naylor, 1991) applied the same paradigm, rCBF measured during orthographic task performance, to a new sample of 83 adults whose reading and IQ test performance had been carefully evaluated in childhood. (More detail on this sample and its adult behavioral outcome is presented in Felton, Naylor and Wood, 1990). Seventy-two were male; seven were left handed and six were ambidextrous (cf. Briggs and Nebes, 1975). This sample permitted not only a replication of the relationship between left temporal flow and task accuracy (in a group with widely varying reading histories) but also a study of the impact of childhood dyslexia on adult brain functioning.

Assignment of subjects to childhood reading levels was by a reading quotient computed independently of IQ (Boder and Jarrico, 1982) using cutoff scores on the WRAT Reading (Jastak and Bijou, 1946) and Gray Oral Reading (Gray, 1955) tests in childhood. Less than or equal to a standard score of 82 on both defined 33 subjects with a classification of reading disabled (RD). Scores on both reading tests above 91 assigned 23 subjects a classification of non-reading disabled (NRD). All of the remaining 27 subjects, unclassifiable as either RD or NRD, were classified as borderline (BL). All were in good physical health and free of psychopathology.

In the first analysis, we were able to replicate the relationship between task accuracy and left hemisphere blood flow in subjects with a broad range of childhood reading ability. As in the normal adult group, task performance significantly predicted flow only at the left superior temporal detector. Further, the effect was independent of age, IQ, gender, years of education, state anxiety, or handedness. The relationship of language activation to the left temporal area is a reliable and replicable one.

In a further analysis, using early reading ability as a predictor of cortical activation, we found that good versus poor childhood readers differed significantly in activation of the temporal lobe site (Wernicke's area). With task accuracy as a covariate, however, group differences in left temporal flow were eliminated — not surprisingly, since poor readers performed the task less well and in both large samples (69 normals and 83 Ortons) good task performance predicted greater left temporal flow.

Our interpretation of the Ojemann model, however, predicts that RDs will show not only less activation in the left temporal area, but also more activation in a nearby, possibly a posterior, site. The prediction proved accurate in that a significant *inverse* relationship was found between childhood reading level and blood flow measured at the angular gyrus. That is, RD subjects had higher angular gyrus flow than either the BL or NRD groups. Just as with the previous finding, statistically equating subjects for childhood verbal and performance IQ, education, age, gender, and state anxiety failed to eliminate the effect. But in contrast to the previous analysis, task accuracy as a covariate also failed to eliminate the effect: good and poor performers both showed elevations of angular gyrus flow, compared to normals. High angular gyrus flow of RDs was also independent of adult reading improvement, where improvement is defined by comparing child and adult scores on the same two oral reading tests that had been used in assigning childhood reading level.

The fact that angular gyrus excess, in dyslexics compared to controls, is independent of task accuracy and reading improvements is challenging. It seems that the only plausible interpretation is to infer a neurobehavioral reorganization that has occurred by the time that childhood reading scores are taken (since they predict the adult angular gyrus excess). At the same time, it must then also be inferred that subsequent learning (as measured by adult reading scores) or other acquired skills (as measured on the orthographic task) do not alter this reorganization.

As described above, the microscopic anomalies observed in the dyslexic left hemisphere could in principle induce altered neural connectivity, hence altered organization. Such re-routing after selective lesions is known in the animal literature (Sur, Garraghty, and Roe, 1988; Frost, 1988). The relocation of embryonic axons would thus constitute true structural displacement, prenatally determined, preventing the development of fully normal language functions. However, since the "displaced" activity of the angular gyrus was related to childhood reading level and not improvement itself or to task accuracy, we would have to posit that only some subset of functions evoked by the task — those not related to task accuracy — are involved in this "relocation."

Although the correlation between left temporal flow and task accuracy suggests that the overall summation of left temporal activity is task related, little detailed specification is possible regarding which types of processes, during the measurement period, are contributing most heavily to the total blood flow activity measure. For example, if the major feature of interest is assumed to be largely perceptual, then the question becomes: does the neural activity involved in correctly rejecting a five letter word imply the same linguistic/orthographic processing as required for a "hit" of a four letter word? If so, then neural activity during a correct rejection should make as great a contribution to the total blood flow score at any given probe site as is made by the neural activity during a hit. (In this case, by definition, any presumed motor component would be having little effect.) By contrast, if the relevant neural activity is largely involved in selective attention to the target, and less attention to the foil, then the difference between neural response to targets and neural response to foils should be the major feature of interest.

While a rough measure of these possible features might be estimated from separate correlations between blood flow and hits and between blood flow and false alarms, a finer approach to the question would be obtainable if a supplementary measure of neural activation could be separately recorded for each trial. Obviously, electrophysiological techniques, while leaving the issue of source generation a matter of debate, are the only suitable ones for such a trial by trial analysis.

As a large N study to characterize major sources of variance in the multivariate space that relates to left temporal functioning, the above study is a useful first step. However, it leaves new questions for future studies. Questions of anatomical, including sub-cortical, detail are addressable by PET. Critical also, however, is the issue of relatively poor temporal resolution, requiring the summation of all neural activity over time — 11 minutes for the Xenon method and 40 minutes for PET studies. In both cases, the "image" sums all of the blood flow or metabolic activity that occurs during the measurement period.

Clearly, the answer to this dilemma is to undertake electrophysiological and metabolism recordings simultaneously, during task performance. This actually is easier with PET than with Xenon blood flow, since the glucose uptake procedure is separate from the actual imaging procedure in PET, whereas in Xenon blood flow task performance is carried on simultaneously with the measurement of radioactivity by externally placed scalp detectors, creating obvious logistical problems.

Another issue has to do with the generality of the orthographic analysis task to the fundamental phonemic processing disorder that is widely discerned in dyslexia. There is clear face validity to the task, of course, but whether it actually taps the more restricted phonemic processing deficit — known from behavioral studies to characterize dyslexia — is still uncertain. Accordingly, a more narrowly circumscribed task, burdening only the perception of fast formant transitions would be desirable. A PET procedure designed to investigate phonemic perception *per se*, would then allow not only a spatially more resolute study but also a study focused on a more circumscribed task.

An important preliminary question is whether there is a blood flow correlate of task performance on a phoneme perception (syllable discrimination) task. That is important, so the results can be compared to those obtained with the orthographic task. This can be addressed by a preliminary study with normals, to characterize the correlation between temporal lobe activity and phoneme discrimination. In line with the principle discussed above, we might well expect that this relatively automatized task could actually be inversely correlated. Poor performers, who are less automatized, might be expected to show additional effort and, therefore, higher flow.

Experiment 3

Exploratory study to define the correlation of rCBF with phonemic task accuracy.

rCBF was measured in a subset of the subjects from Experiments 1 and 2 — 29 male subjects with no evidence of reading problems or language delay and 18 reading disabled subjects. Phonemic stimuli were six consonant-vowel syllables (/da/, /ba/, /pa/, /ga/, /ka/, /ta/), synthesized on a Bliss system at Brown University. Subjects listened to these at the rate of one each 2.5 sec, responding with a button press to the /da/ target which occurred a random 1/6 of the time. Each stimulus was 250 ms long, 40 ms of which contained the distinguishing formant transition. To avoid ceiling effects, stimuli were embedded in speech babble (indistinguishable noise containing speech frequencies) such that on preliminary tests subjects free of language disability made 80% correct responses. Accuracy was again defined as d-prime. No feedback was given during data collection. The task lasted approximately nine minutes, during rCBF tracer inhalation and clearance.

Behaviorally, normals and RDs did not differ on this task either with respect to accuracy or speed of responding; neither were they distinguished by differences in blood flow at any given site. However, in the normal subjects alone, higher task accuracy predicted lower flow at the left superior temporal site ($p = 0.02$). Clearly, this is exactly the inverse of the orthographic task finding. In contrast, RD subjects alone showed a trend toward *greater* left temporal flow with better task performance.

Thus, normal adults reduce left temporal activation during discrimination of phonemes, but enhance the same location when analyzing whole words. From our previous logic, we interpret this as a difference between the highly automatized processing of basic auditory code (phonemes) for which the temporal substrate is highly evolved and the more novel process of counting the number of letters in a whole word. The RD subjects seem to respond differently, though they perform the task adequately. Indeed, the trend in dyslexics is for an increase in cortical activation with good performance on the task. For the disabled reader, then, the task is within grasp (given adquate time) but it is not automatic. Furthermore, the left temporal area is excitable, not silent.

Experiment 4

Simultaneous PET and auditory evoked response measures during phonemic task performance.

In this exploratory study, the same phonetic discrimination stimuli were employed in ten RD subjects from Exp. 3 and ten normal controls, using PET methodology and simultaneously recording auditory evoked responses (AERs).

Regional brain activity was imaged with a positron emission tomograph using ^{18}F-2-deoxyglucose (FDG) as the radioactive tracer, with quality assurance procedures confirming radiochemical purity and pharmaceutical quality. In-plane resolution was 7.6 mm and z-dimension resolution was 10.9 mm. FDG was introduced by way of an intravenous saline drip, started in advance to allow time for subjects to overcome any anxiety due to the needle stick. Nine planes, parallel to the canthomeatal line, were done 40 minutes after injection. The dependent measure, rate of glucose metabolism, was calculated according to Sokoloff et al. (1977). Axial magnetic resonance images provided a template for locating PET regions of interest.

Simultaneous with FDG uptake, AERs were measured using a 32-electrode montage with a linked-ear reference. A sampling rate of 200 counts per second (5 ms) extended over a 320 ms epoch. Three components, positive components at 120 ms and 200 ms and a negative component at 160 ms, were identified by visual inspection of the data. The dependent measures were the amplitudes in microvolts (referenced to each subject's average baseline) at each latency.

During the 40 minutes of glucose uptake, in a darkened, soundproof, electrically shielded room, subjects listened to strings of six computer generated stop consonant-vowel syllables (as described in Experiment 3) separated by two seconds and were instructed to respond with a button-push each time the "target" /da/ was heard (25% of the time, randomly distributed). Five-minute trials, usually six per subject, continued until uptake was complete. Hits, misses, false alarms, and correct rejections were counted, but no feedback was given. AERs for each behavioral condition were averaged separately. Perfect performance would have yielded averaged AERs to 240 hits or to 714 correct rejections for each subject. Normals performed more accurately than RDs, perhaps because of the time constraints and the 40-minute long task duration.

The normal and RD groups were examined separately to discover if the PET and AER profiles resembled the blood flow findings relating left temporal neural activity and task accuracy, i.e., an inverse correlation in the normal group and a positive correlation in the RD group. In normal subjects, the PET glucose measure in the central peri-Sylvian area (both temporal and fronto-parietal) showed a uniform trend toward negative Spearman correlations with d-prime. This was significant at $p = 0.03$ in a one-tailed (a priori) test, at the supra-Sylvian site immediately above Heschl's gyrus.

Of additional interest in normals is the significant negative Spearman correlation between d-prime and the left and right central segments of the anterior corpus callosum. These correlations (−0.90 and −0.82, $p < 0.0005$ and $p < 0.005$, respectively) were the strongest of any in the brain. White matter glucose measurements with PET are of particular interest: because of the possibility of axoplasmic transport they could index activity in upstream gray matter cortical sites; and, because they are concentrated in such a narrow region (analogous to the neck of a funnel), they may index the upstream activity far more sensitively than would local measurements made directly in the cortex.

The correlation between AERs and task accuracy in the normal group is also provocative. At a latency of 120 ms, a positive component (P1) measured at C3 (between top center and the mid-temporal lobe by the International 10—20 System) was significantly ($p = < 0.01$) negatively correlated (Spearman) with task accuracy (d-prime). As would be expected from a left, centrally recorded component believed to reflect direct linguistic/perceptual processing (Wood et al., 1971), the correlations are equally strong for this component measured on correct hit trials and on correct rejection trials. Consistent with the above-described inverse correlation between d-prime and the anterior callosal glucose measure, P1 at

C3 is correlated positively with anterior corpus callosum glucose ($p = 0.04$, one-tailed).

In the RD group, there was a positive correlation between task accuracy and PET glucose utilization in a circumscribed region on the superior temporal lobe, corresponding approximately to the more lateral half to two-thirds of Heschl's gyrus. It is notable that left temporal planum glucose utilization was positively related ($p = 0.04$, one-tailed) to P1 amplitude. That makes it all the more instructive that this left temporal lobe activity — whether indexed by glucose utilization or by the P1 component at C3 — is unrelated to task accuracy in dyslexics. Interestingly, there was also a suggestion (at $p = 0.06$, two-tailed) that the C3/P1 component was negatively correlated with anterior corpus callosum PET glucose measures, corroborating the glucose-accuracy correlation.

Of special significance is the fact that all the correlations involving the AER P120 at C3 are of highly similar strength and statistical significance both for trials on which a hit occurred and for trials on which a correct rejection occurred. Thus, it is the more purely perceptual aspect of the task — requiring the same phonemic processing for a hit as well as a correct rejection — that is being measured.

Observations from Experiments 3 and 4 together, albeit based on relatively small numbers of subjects, can be summarized as follows.

1. When discriminating target phonemes accurately, normal subjects show diminished blood flow, hence deactivation, in the region of the left temporal lobe detector (in contrast to the positive correlation between temporal flow and accuracy that had earlier been obtained with the orthographic task).
2. PET measures of glucose utilization conform to the same general trend: peri-Sylvian cortex tends to have less activity in normals during accurate task performance than during inaccurate performance. This inverse relationship is especially pronounced in the anterior corpus callosum.
3. In contrast to normals, dyslexics performing most accurately show the greatest levels of glucose utilization in the vicinity of Heschl's gyrus.
4. The P1 auditory evoked potential, during the PET glucose uptake, follows the same trend as the glucose utilization findings and the earlier rCBF findings. Furthermore, the relationship holds during correct rejections as much as during correct hits, thus suggesting the more purely perceptual aspects of the task are the most relevant.

One interpretation of the above findings is then that in normals, accurate processing of speech sounds is so well automatized that it ordinarily requires minimal cortical activation. Indeed, greater activation in normals signals inaccurate and correspondingly effortful processing. Conversely, if the task is inherently poorly automatized in dyslexics, for reasons of chronic phonemic processing disorder, then left cerebral activation becomes necessary for accurate task performance — hence the positive correlation.

To be sure, the above conclusions on 10 normals and 10 dyslexics are necessarily tentative. Some of them depend on one-tailed tests, using assumptions from prior studies; so more definitive, larger N studies are clearly in order. Their value is perhaps more methodological than definitively empirical: they illustrate a set of issues that will need to be faced in the larger studies.

SUMMARY

From an empirical point of view, the above experiments present interesting data that bear upon the hypothesized left temporal substrate for developmental dyslexia. These might conveniently be summarized as showing (a) posterior displacement, from the superior temporal lobe to the angular gyrus, in dyslexics, when the activating task requires orthographic analysis of auditorially perceived words; (b) the contrast, in normals, between positive correlations of left temporal flow with orthographic task accuracy and negative correlations of left temporal flow with phonemic discrimination accuracy; and (c) the perceptual (distinct from motoric or relevance-related) nature of the phenomena being measured.

As the above review makes clear, the investigation of left temporal abnormality in dyslexia, through functional neuroimaging techniques, presents distinctive methodological issues. They can be summarized in the form of cautions for the study of left temporal dysfunction in dyslexia, as follows:

1. Assumptions about the relationship between task accuracy and the locus and direction of metabolic change during task performance are unwarrented. In particular, it is a necessary preliminary empirical question what the locus and direction of such changes should be. In this case, orthographic task accuracy is positively related to left temporal flow in normals, but phonemic task accuracy is negatively related. This finding suggests the importance of automaticity and other dimensions of difference between tasks. It cannot be assumed that subcomponents of a given task that is positively correlated with task accuracy will themselves be positively correlated. In a more general sense, here is a trap for the unwary researcher who relies too heavily on subtraction logic (as though a given task could only have components in it that are positively summing to its overall metabolic impact).

2. It cannot be assumed that similar mechanisms or similar loci of functional activation should characterize a normal and a dyslexic group. In this case, it appears that the brains of dyslexics function in a rather

different way from normals on a phonemic discrimination task (indeed, as they had also functioned differently on the orthographic analysis task in the blood flow experiment).

3. Because of the above two problems, comparisons of mean activity at some brain location between a normal and a dyslexic group during the performance of a relevant task may be completely uninterpretable until the multivariate structure of individual differences, relating task accuracy to the locus and intensity of brain activation, is characterized.

4. It should not be assumed that large blocks of neural tissue (such as "left versus right" or "anterior versus posterior") function as single units. According to these data, not only is the "temporal lobe" a vast collection of separately functioning parts, so even is the superior temporal gyrus. Whereas the rCBF studies could resolve no further than a circle of two and a half or three centimeters in diameter, PET can resolve regions substantially smaller than that, and it is instructive that only a narrow focus in the left superior temporal lobe — corresponding to the lateral aspect of Heschl's gyrus — is found to be positively related to task accuracy in dyslexics. It is, of course, theoretically instructive that the dyslexic deficit should show up as excess activation limited to the region of Heschl's gyrus; but whatever the theoretical import of the finding, its methodological significance is to support fractionation of cortical areas so that finer grained analyses can be undertaken.

5. Unidimensional physiological studies are, as the above review demonstrates, risky. If any one of the above methods had been relied upon exclusively for conclusions about abnormal temporal lobe function in dyslexia, interpretive mistakes might well have been made. For example, the inverse correlation between left temporal flow and phonemic discrimination accuracy in normals — derived from the rCBF technique — may be limited to a more circumscribed area in or near Heschl's gyrus. On the other hand, if PET alone had been used, we could have had no confidence that the total summed activity, during task performance, reflected perceptual processing both on the hits as well as on the correct rejections. Absent an electrophysiological measurement, from a site believed to reflect superior temporal processing, it would have been difficult to know which parts of task performance were most related to the total glucose utilization value for the entire period, for a given location. On the other hand, electrophysiological measurements by themselves present considerable difficulty in source localization.

In conclusion, we offer the above review as a methodological starting point for further investigations in dyslexia research. What it suggests, more than anything else, is that subsequent progress may well be facilitated by: studies that contrast the multivariate brain activation structure of a normal sample with that of a dyslexic sample, by careful isolation of small brain regions to take advantage of PET methodology, and by multi-dimensional rather than unidimensional converging operations, capitalizing on the different spatial and temporal resolutions of the different physiological methods.

ACKNOWLEDGMENT

Supported by Grant No. HD-21887 from the United States Public Health Service to Bowman Gray School of Medicine, Winston-Salem, NC.

REFERENCES

Boder, E., and Jarrico, S. (1982). *The Boder Test of Reading-Spelling Patterns: A Diagnostic Screening Test for Subtypes of Reading Disability.* New York: Grune and Stratton.

Briggs, G. G. and Nebes, R. D. (1975). Patterns of hand preference in a student population. *Cortex, 11,* 230—238.

Duane, D. D. (1989). Commentary on dyslexia and neurodevelopmental pathology. *Journal of Learning Disabilities, 22,* 219—220.

Felton, R. H. and Wood, F. B. (1989). Cognitive deficits in reading disability and attention deficit disorder. *Journal of Learning Disabilities, 1,* 3—13.

Felton, R. H., Naylor, C. E. and Wood, F. B. (1990). The neuropsychological profile of adult dyslexics. *Brain and Language, 39,* 485—497.

Flowers, D. L., Wood, F. B., and Naylor, C. E. (1991). Regional cerebral blood flow correlates of language processes in adult dyslexics. *Archives of Neurology, 48,* 637—643.

Frost, D. O. (1988). Mechanisms of structural and functional development in the thalamus: Retinal projections to the auditory and somatosensory systems in normal and experimentally manipulated hamsters. *In* M. Bentivoglio and R. Spreafico (Eds.), *Cellular thalamic mechanisms.* Amsterdam: Elsevier (pp. 447—464).

Galaburda, A. M., Sherman, G. F., Rosen, G. D., Aboitiz, F., and Geschwind, N. (1985). Developmental dyslexia: four consecutive patients with cortical anomalies. *Annals of Neurology, 18,* 222—233.

Galaburda, A. M. and Steinmetz. 1991. This publication.

Goldman, P. S. (1978). Neuronal plasticity in primate telencephalon: Anomalous projections induced by prenatal removal of frontal cortex. *Science, 202,* 768—770.

Goldman-Rakic, P. S. and Rakic, P. (1984). Experimentally modified convolutional patterns in non-human primates: Possible relevance of connections to cerebral dominance in humans. In N. Geschwind and A. M. Galaburda (Eds.), *Biological Foundation of Cerebral Dominance.* Cambridge, MA: Harvard University Press.

Gray, W. S. (1955). *Standardized Oral Reading Paragraphs.* Indianapolis: Bobbs-Merrill.

Green, D. M. and Swets, J. (1966). *Signal Detection Theory.* New York: Wiley Press.

Jastak, J. and Bijou, S. (1946). *Wide Range Achievement Test.* Wilmington: Jastak Associates.

Kaufman, W. E. and Galaburda, A. M. (1989). Cerebrocortical microdysgenesis in neurologically normal subjects: A histopathologic study. *Neurology, 39,* 238—244.

Larsen, J. P., Hoien, T., Lundberg, I. and Odegaard, H. (1990). MRI evaluation of the size and symmetry of the planum temporale in adolescents with developmental dyslexia. *Brain and Language, 39,* 289—301.

Ojemann, G. A. (1983). Brain organization for language from the perspective of electrial stimulation mapping. *The Behavioral and Brain Sciences, 6,* 189—230.

Ojemann, G. A. and Whitaker, H. A. (1978). Language localization and variability. *Brain and Language, 6,* 239—260.

Pennington, B. F., Lefly, D. L., Van Orden, G. C., Bookman, M. O. and Smith, S. D. (1987). Is phonology bypassed in normal or dyslexic development? *Annals of Dyslexia, 37,* 62—89.

Prohovnik, I., Knudson, E., and Risberg, J. (1985). Theoretical evaluation and stimulation test of the inital slope index for uninvasive rCBF. In H. Hartman and S. Hoyer (Eds.), *Cerebral Blood Flow &Metabolism Measurement.* Berlin: Springer-Verlag.

Rasmussen, T., and Milner, B. (1977). The role of early left-brain injury in determining lateralizations of cerebral speech functions. *Annals of the New York Academy of Science, 299,* 355—369.

Sokoloff, L., Reivich, M., Kennedy, C., DesRosiers, M. H., Patlak, C. S., Pettigrew, K. D., Sakurada, O. and Shiniohara, M. (1977). The [14C] deoxyglucose method for the measurement of local cerebral glucose utilization: Theory, procedure, and normal values in the conscious and anesthetized albino rat. *Journal of Neurochemistry, 28,* 897—916.

Spielberger, C. D., Gorsuch, R. L., Luchene, R., Vagg, P. R. and Jacobs, G. A. (1983). *Manual for the State-Trait Anxiety Inventory (STAI) — Form Y.* Palo Alto, CA, Consulting Psychology Press.

Sur, M., Garraghty, P. E. and Roe, A. W. (1988). Experimentally induced visual projections into auditory thalamus and cortex. *Science, 242,* 1437—1440.

Vellutino, F. R. (1979). *Dyslexia: Theory and research.* Cambridge, MA: MIT Press.

Wood, C. C., Goff, W. R. and Say, R. S. (1971). Auditory evoked potentials during speech perception. *Science, 173,* 1248—1251.

Wood, F. (1980). Theoretical, methodological, and statistical implications of the inhalation regional cerebral blood flow technique for the study of brain-behavior relationships. *Brain and Language, 9,* 1—8.

Wood, F. B. (1983). Laterality of cerebral function: Its investigation by measurement of localized brain activity. In J. Hellige (Ed.), *Cerebral Function and Asymmetry: Method, Theory and Application.* New York: Praeger.

Wood, F. (1990). Functional neuroimaging in neurobehavioral research. In A. A. Boulton, G. B. Baker and M. Hiscock (Eds.), *Neuromethods: Neuropsychology.* Clifton, New Jersey: Humana Press, pp. 107—125.

Wood, F. and Felton, R. H. (1983). Physiological specification of the phenotype in genetic language disorders: Prospects for the use of indicators of localized brain metabolism. In C. L. Ludlow and J. A. Cooper (Eds.), *Genetic aspects of speech and language disorders.* New York: Academic Press, pp. 53—69.

Cerebral Laterality in Dyslexic Children: Implications for Phonological Word Decoding Deficits

JOHN KERSHNER and JOHN MICALLEF
Ontario Institute for Studies in Education 252 Bloor St. West Toronto, Ontario, Canada M5S 1V6

ABSTRACT: The study evaluated a substantially updated version of Orton's (1937) "classical" idea of a significant relatonship in dyslexic children between cerebral lateralization and their word decoding deficits. Attentional lateralization was examined under the assumption that covert spatial attention when directed contralaterally interacts with age-invariant cerebral asymmetries for receptive speech. Thirty dysphonetic dyslexic children were compared to 30 younger normal readers who were matched to the dyslexics in reading comprehension. The children were tested in left ear (LE) and right ear (RE) directed attention dichotic listening (DAD), and in pseudoword decoding, word recognition, reading comprehension, spelling, arithmetic, and in general intelligence (IQ). Group comparisons in DAD failed to show any differences, confirming the mounting evidence that dyslexia is not related to incomplete lateralization. Entering the DAD scores of the dyslexics (LE first, LE second, RE first, RE second) as predictors of achievement revealed that, independently of chronological age (CA) and IQ, their ability to recall items from the LE first produced a negative regression which predicted 42 percent of the variance in pseudoword decoding. Selective report from the LE also produced small but significant negative correlations with visual recognition of real words and spelling; but no relationship to reading comprehension. IQ was related to reading comprehension and to the ability to shift attention from the LE to the RE. Eventhough the dyslexics were lateralized normally, weak lateralization was related specifically to phonological word decoding, a core deficit in dyslexia. However, unlike Orton's concept, these findings suggest that dyslexics suffer from exuberant right hemisphere processing in response to spatial attentional demands that, in turn, interferes transcallosally with the development of the sound-symbol representations that are required for fluent reading. Lateralization, per se, is unaffected by the disorder.

KEYWORDS: dyslexia, lateralization, attention, dichotic listening, word recognition, reading.

INTRODUCTION

In his remarkably prescient and influential Salmon Lecture[1], Orton (1937) was among the first to identify a failure in single word recognition as "the hallmark" of developmental dyslexia. Mounting experimental evidence substantiating this clinical observation suggests in addition that an insensitivity to the phonological attributes of printed words lies at the core of the disability (Liberman and Shankweiler, 1979; Stanovich, 1988; Vellutino, 1979; Vellutino, Scanlon and Tanzman, 1990). This increasingly concensual theoretical and definitional viewpoint may prove to be instru-

Reading and Writing: An Interdisciplinary Journal 3: 395—411, 1991.
© 1991 *Kluwer Academic Publishers.*

mental in the development of a cohesive pool of basic research and in educational interventions (Berninger and Traweek, 1990).

In the same lecture, which summarized a decade of intensive research into childhood language disorders, Orton (1937) concluded with the now-classical theme that such word decoding problems may be the result of neurophysiological deviations in the process of developing unilateral linguistic superiority of the left cerebral hemisphere over the right. In contrast to the demonstrated centrality of word decoding deficits to dyslexia, this latter theoretical proposition on the neuropsychology of the disorder has not received any clear-cut empirical support. However, although recent data have disconfirmed the developmental implications and the interhemispheric mechanics of Orton's original model, Bryden (1988) on a note of guarded optimism suggested that dyslexia may be linked to some modified version of Orton's original conceptualization. Thus, Orton may have been correct in claiming a fundamental relationship between cerebral lateralization and dyslexia.

The present study was designed to test a qualified version of Orton's lateralization hypothesis. Both Kershner (1988) and Obrzut (1988) have suggested that developmental reading disorders may be produced by an interhemispheric attentional dysfunction interacting with age-invariant cerebral asymmetries. Left hemisphere specialization for linguistic processing remains constant with age and across reading ability groups; whereas lateralized attentional abilities develop during the early school years (Anderson and Hugdahl, 1987; Geffen and Wale, 1979) and differentiate children with dyslexia from age-matched controls (Kershner, 1988; Obrzut, 1988). Also see Gladstone and Best (1985) for a similar theoretical argument.

These ideas have been refined in two recent directed attention, dichotic listening (DAD) experiments (Kershner and Morton, 1990). According to Bryden (1988) the DAD procedure is the preferred method for measuring the lateralization of receptive speech in dyslexic children. Dichotic listening, which requires the immediate recall of different competing verbal stimuli that are projected simultaneously over stereo headphones to both ears, has been carried out usually in a free-recall format. A right ear advantage (REA) or difference in performance between the LE and the RE is an indication of the linguistic superiority of the left cerebral hemisphere. The DAD modification requires exclusive surveillance and report from each ear in a predetermined sequence. Thus, the DAD paradigm controls for ambient fluctuations of attention in estimates of lateralization, i.e., the REA, and, at the same time, provides four ear by attending-order measures (LE first, LE second, RE first, RE second) of the interaction of lateral attention with cerebral asymmetries. The validity of inferring intra-hemispheric and inter-hemispheric attentional processes from DAD is based on two principal lines of evidence. First is the knowledge that laterally displaced attention challenges attentional activation mechanisms in the contralateral hemisphere (Kinsbourne, 1970). Secondly, reallocating attention across the vertical meridian is known to implicate the neurological structures of the corpus callosum and the interplay of processes between hemispheres (Reuter-Lorenz and Fendrich, 1990).

Using DAD with two different cohorts of reading disabled children, Kershner and Morton (1990) found that the disabled children produced REAs that were equal in magnitude to groups of age-matched normal readers. However, the disabled children had greater difficulty than controls when they were forced to spatially orient their attention covertly (eye and head movements were controlled to the center of the visual field) in specific ear-order combinations. The reading impaired children were poorer in DAD recall when the LE (first and second) was precued for selective report. They were also inferior in shifting attention from the LE first to the RE second. No group differences emerged at the RE first, which presumably depends relatively less on the inter-hemispheric coordination of attention with language. These results suggested that dyslexia may involve an incompatibility between right hemisphere attentional control and left hemisphere language. Additionally, the data suggested mutually interfering consequences for both. For instance, when the dyslexics were directed left their overall performance was significantly depressed and their ability to recall from the LE was reduced disproportionately to the smaller increase of intrusions from the RE. The dyslexics' inability to reorient to the RE second was interpreted as a failure to engage the left hemisphere following right hemisphere activation. Thus, the Kershner and Morton (1990) results suggest that some of the linguistic deficits in dyslexia may result from a right hemisphere attentional dysfunction which interferes with the efficient development of left hemisphere language capabilities.

Notably, although children with dyslexia appear not to differ from good readers in cerebral asymmetries, Orton may have been correct in associating the strength of their lateralization to the severity of the handicap. According to this attentionally-based modification of the Ortonian claim, dyslexics who are relatively better at attending left (reducing their lateralization), paradoxically, should demonstrate more severe word recognition deficits. By the same reasoning, their ability to shift attentional processing from the LE to the RE (increasing their lateralization) should facilitate their word recognition ability. Therefore, while we do not expect group differences in lateralization, we predict that, unlike normal readers, weak lateralization in dyslexic children will be related to their poor phonological word decoding.

PLAN OF THE STUDY

The purpose of the study was to test for a functional connection in dyslexic children between spatial attentional activation during linguistic processing and specific deficits in phonological word decoding. We tested this prediction in an orthogonally-balanced, DAD paradigm using correlational and regression analyses to compare dyslexics with a group of younger, normal readers who were matched with the dyslexics in reading comprehension.

Originally, we had included an age-matched control group; but a ceiling effect on the dichotic listening task precluded them from the study. Nevertheless, a reading level-matched comparison group using multiple regression techniques gives us a strong test of our hypothesis (Mamen, Ferguson and Backman, 1986). For example, in addition to controlling for reading experience, we anticipated equivalent lateralization between groups in this design because the REA does not change with age or differ reliably in the absence of attentional bias betwen dyslexics and normal readers (Obrzut, 1988). Moreover, because children prior to eight years of age have difficulty directing their attention to the left ear (Geffen and Wale, 1979) and shifting from left to right in dichotic recall (Kershner and Chyczij, in preparation), we expected dichotic performance in each ear-order condition to be equivalent. Relative difficulties in attending left and shifting right when digit strings are used as stimuli are characteristics of dichotic listening performance that older dyslexic children appear to have in common with younger normal readers. Thus, any group differences in the power of the dichotic task to predict performance on the criterion measures should not result from ability differences in either dichotic listening or in absolute levels of reading comprehension.

This is the first DAD study with digits to use a within-subjects design for the two ear Orders. But, it is particularly significant that the present study examines the possibility that maladaptive linguistic lateralization in dyslexics may be related specifically to their phonological word processing deficits. To explore this issue thoroughtly, we included measures of pseudoword decoding, word recognition, reading comprehension, spelling, arithmetic, and IQ.

METHOD

Subjects and Criterion Measures

Thirty right-handed male dyslexic children, mean chronological age (CA) = 11.3 years, SD = 1.1, were selected from a larger pool of approximately 500 learning disabled childredn (LD) in the largest school board in Canada. Initially, all of the LD children had been identified by a Special Education Identification, Placement and Review Committee (SEIPRC) according to Ontario Ministry of Education Guidelines. From this larger school population, school psychologists and LD teachers were asked to recommend individual children based on a list of stringent criteria: (1) in a special LD program but not in a language disability class; (2) right-handed and male caucasian between 7—12 years of age; (3) assessed for IQ on the Wechsler Intelligence Scale for Children-Revised (WISC-R) (Wechsler, 1974) within the last two years with Performance IQ ⩾ 90; (4) audiometric screening showing normal pure-tone thresholds bilaterally at 20 dB (A) (250—8,000 Hz); (5) no apparent visual-spatial problems; (6) no neurological impairment; (7) no atypical absences from school; (8) no English as a second language problems; (9) no general motivational problems; (10) healthy and not on prescription medication; (11) no evidence of primary emotional problems; (12) not attention deficit disordered or hyperactive; (13) not economically deprived; (14) clear evidence of a severe disability in phonics. As children were recommended by the psychology staff and LD teachers as potential subjects, they entered a second screening stage in which they were individually tested on the Woodcock Word Attack Test-Revised (Woodcock, 1987), a measure of pseudoword decoding which is heavily dependent on phonology. If they scored ⩽ the 17th percentile by age in pseudoword decoding, they were accepted into the study and given the remaining criterion tests. These were the Woodcock Test of Passage Comprehension-Revised (Woodcock, 1987), and the Wide Range Achievement Test (WRAT) (Jastak and Wilkinson, 1984) — Reading (word recognition), Spelling, and Arithmetic.

As dyslexic children entered the study, the staff at the same schools were given a second set of criteria to recommend children for the reading level-matched normal group. Based on the grade-level reading comprehension scores of the dyslexics, thirty right-handed caucasian male normal children, mean CA = 7.8, SD = 0.9, were selected from grades one to four. They had to show at least average achievement in school, especially in reading. As such normal children were recommended, they were given all of the criterion tests and only approved if they scored ⩾ the 25th percentile on each test. Finally, they were accepted into the study if they were able to score ⩾ 90 in IQ, based on derived Verbal and Performance IQs that were calculated from individually administered Vocabulary and Block Design subtests from the WISC-R.

Dichotic Materials

The tape of dichotic digits were designed by P. Henninger and recorded at the Bryden Laboratory, the University of Waterloo, Ontario. Stimuli of 350 msec duration were produced from a computer tape of digitized natural speech (adult female voice) after amplitude and duration normalization. A total of 64 dichotic pairs of monosyllable digits was arranged into 16 trials consisting of two blocks (8 trials each) of quadruple pairs.

They were presented at the rate of 2 pairs per sec within trials and a 14 sec intertrial interval. The dichotic tape was played on a TEAC 160 Stereo Cassette Deck-C47, through Realistic NOVA 40 headphones. A Hewlett-Packard 427A voltmeter was used to measure output at each headphone. The ambient noise level was 30dB. The average signal amplitude for each channel at each outlet was 70 dB.

Dichotic Procedures

Dichotic testing was done individually in a quiet room in two sessions separated by a one to two-week interval. Half of the children in session one were assigned to a LE first Order and half were assigned to a RE first Order. In the second testing session the Orders were reversed so that each child obtained a LE and a RE score in both Orders. Performance at each of the four ear-order conditions (LE first, LE second, RE first, RE second) was scored for the number of correct digits from the attended channel and the number of intrusions from the unattended channel. Testing was preceded by eight warmup trials of quadruple digit pairs presented in a free-recall format. The children were instructed to keep their head forward and to fixate their eyes throughout the testing on a yellow dot that was placed 60 cm in front of them at eye level. A research assistant who was blind to the experimental hypotheses sat behind the visual fixation card to record the children's oral responses and to monitor eye movements. The children were instructed to report the numbers heard only from the designated ear. They were asked to report four digits per trial, and the target ear was touched by the assistant and by the children. If they were unsure, guessing was encouraged. In each ordered session, following eight trials from one ear they were instructed to switch their attention to the other ear for eight trials. Again, the target ear was touched by the assistant and by the children. Headsets were reversed between the directed conditions to offset any channel differences in signal-to-noise ratio.

This procedure produced a Reading Level (Dyslexic, Normal) by Order (LE first, RE first) by Session (One, Two) by Directed Instructions (Directed Left, Directed right) by Ear (LE, RE) research design with repeated measures on the last four factors.

RESULTS

Sample Characteristics

Table 1 displays the means (Ms) and standard deviations (SDs) for the dyslexics and normal readers on the WISC-R and on the criterion meas-

Table 1. Means and standard deviations for the Dyslexic and Normals for age and IQ

	Dyslexics Mean	SD	Normals Mean	SD
Age in Years	11.3	1.1	7.8	0.9
Verbal IQ[a]	85.6	9.1	108.5	10.9
Performance IQ[a]	102.2	9.7	111.3	12.7
Word Attack[b]:				
raw score	12.4	6.0	20.1	8.4
standard score	69.5	13.5	102.7	9.2
Passage Comprehension[b]				
raw score	25.4*	8.0	27.3*	8.4
standard score	71.5	9.6	103.9	8.6
Reading[c]				
raw score	44.2	10.9	56.1	10.6
standard score	66.9	10.3	102.8	9.6
Spelling[c]				
raw score	24.3	11.3	34.5	7.0
standard score	66.3	7.0	100.3	12.7
Arithmetic[c]				
raw score	23.3*	3.9	21.1*	3.4
standard score	76.9	11.3	100.6	11.1

* all group comparisons *except* these are statistically significant, p. < 0.05.
[a] IQ scores are based on the Wechsler Intelligence Scale for Children-Revised.
[b] subtests of the Woodcock Reading Mastery Test-Revised.
[c] subtests of the Wide Range Achievement Test-Revised.

ures. Multiple t tests between groups, after a Bonferoni correction for inflated Type I error, indicated significant differences in CA, Verbal IQ, Performance IQ, and on each academic criterion measure except the raw score comparisons in Passage Comprehension and in WRAT Arithmetic. These results show: (1) that, although the reading groups were matched successfully in raw score Passage Comprehension, the dyslexics remained poorer in raw score Word Attack and WRAT word recognition; (2) the Performance IQ scores of the dyslexics were distributed in the normal range with an average discrepancy of two SDs between their Word Attack scores and intellectual potential. Kolmogorov-Smirnov Goodness of Fit Tests for each group on each measure indicated normal distributions except for the dyslexics' raw scores in WRAT Spelling, $Z = 1.436$, $p < 0.05$. All statistical computations were performed using the standard age scores.

General Laterality Results

The Ms and SDs of the dichotic testing are presented in Table 2. Kolmogorov-Smirnov Tests indicated that no group by condition mean score deviated significantly from normality. Thus, there is no suggestion of ceiling or floor effects in the data. Preliminary analyses indicated that there were no Session or Group by Session effects; so the two Sessions were combined and not considered further. A four-factor, Group by Directed Ear by Order by Ear repeated measures ANOVA on the scores presented on Table 2 revealed only that both groups obtained an REA, $F(1,58) = 179.5$, $p < 0.001$. Entering CA, Performance IQ, and Verbal IQ as covariates did not influence the results. No other effects approached significance, indicating that there were no mean score differences between groups in cerebral asymmetries or in the effects of attention on cerebral lateralization. A tally of the number of subjects with at least a one digit REA confirmed this conclusion. Nearly an equal number of subjects were found with an REA in both reading Groups and in each Order. Sixty-three percent of the dyslexics and sixty-six percent of the normal readers obtained an REA in both orders. Test, retest reliabilities over the two orders were 0.74 for the dyslexics and 0.64 for the normal readers.

Use of the Lambda Index

Pearson Product-Moment correlations between the number of digits

Table 2. Mean percentage of dichotic digits reported for the ordered conditions

	Left Ear First Order		Right Ear First Order	
	LE	RE	LE	RE
Dyslexics, DL				
Mean	59	35	62	33
SD	14	15	12	12
Dyslexics, DR				
Mean	27	68	27	68
SD	11	13	15	15
Normals, DL				
Mean	56	38	58	36
SD	16	15	13	13
Normals, DR				
Mean	26	69	23	71
SD	16	13	11	11

DL = directed left and DR = direct right
LE = left ear and RE = right ear

reported correctly from each attended ear and the intrusions from the unattended ear produced negative correlations in each group at each ear of greater than −0.93, $p < 0.001$. This finding suggests a common attentional mechanism in selecting correct items while inhibiting unattended items and it justifies the use of a data-reduction index to combine the correct and intrusion responses. Consequently, the correlational and regression analyses were performed using the directed attention lambda transformation recommended by Bryden and Sprott (1981). This coefficient yields four directed attention scores for each subject corresponding to each of the ear-order conditions. The lambda ratio of correct responses (C) to intrusions (I) reflects the strength of attending to the precued channel, $(\lambda) = \text{Ln}(C/I)$. A positive directed attention lambda indicates an REA and LEAs are given a negative sign.

Figure 1 shows the similar mean performance of the dyslexics in each ear-order condition after the Cs and Is were combined into directed attention lambda coefficients. Also, there were no notable discrepancies in the SDs. For the dyslexics: LF, SD = 0.77; LS, SD = 0.56; RF, SD = 0.71; RS, RD = 0.83. For the normals: LF, SD = 0.71; LS, SD = 0.63; RF, SD = 0.79; RS, SD = 0.68. Kolmogorov-Smirnov Tests indicated that all group by ear-order lambda scores were distributed normally.

Correlational Results

Table 3 reports Pearson Product-Moment correlations among the criterion variables. The only noteworthy result was that pseudoword decoding

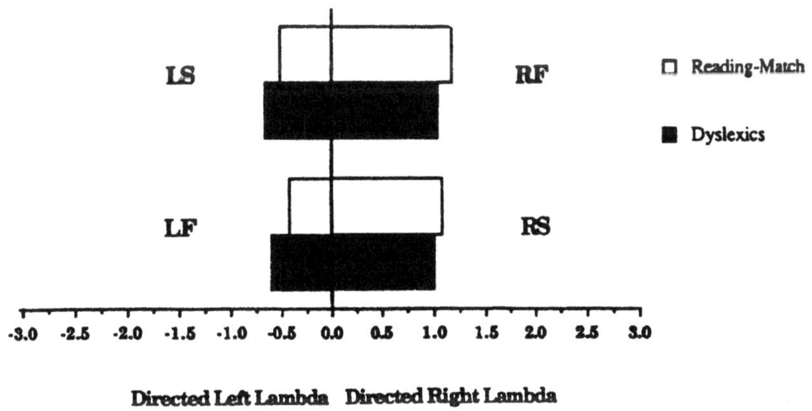

Fig. 1. Mean Directed Attention Lambda Scores Comparing Normals with Dyslexics in the Left Ear First (LF), Left Ear Second (LS), Right Ear First (RF) and Right Ear Second (RS) Orders.

Table 3. Correlations between IQ and the criterion variables for the dyslexics and normals

Measures	Groups	VIQ[a]	PIQ[a]	WWA[b]	WPC[b]	WR[c]	WS[c]
PIQ[a]							
	Dyslexic	0.44**					
	Normals	−0.14					
WWA[b]							
	Dyslexic	0.06	−0.18				
	Normals	0.16	0.07				
WPC[b]							
	Dyslexic	0.42**	0.21	0.15			
	Normals	0.36*	0.04	0.53**			
WR[c]							
	Dyslexic	0.29	0.13	0.51**	0.61**		
	Normals	0.28	−0.04	0.80**	0.69**		
WS[c]							
	Dyslexic	0.31	0.22	0.36*	0.46**	0.62**	
	Normals	0.17	−0.07	0.72**	0.37*	0.72**	
WA[c]							
	Dyslexic	0.15	0.42**	0.08	0.40**	0.18	0.35*
	Normals	0.27	0.11	0.15	−0.09	−0.28	0.36*

* $p < 0.05$.
** $p < 0.01$.
[a] VIQ and PIQ = verbal and performance intelligence on the Wechsler Intelligence Scale for Children-Revised.
[b] WWA and WPC = Word Attack and Passage Comprehension Subtests of the Woodcock Reading Mastery Test-Revised
[c] WR, WS, and WA = Reading, Spelling and Arithmetic Subtests of the Wide Range Achievement Test-Revised.

was related to reading comprehension in the normal readers but not in the dyslexics. The Pearson Product-Moment correlations on Table 4 between the dichotic lambda scores and the criterion measures are crucial to the predictions of the study. The dyslexics produced significant negative correlations in LE recall for Word Attack, WRAT Reading, and WRAT spelling and significant positive correlations between RE second recall and both Verbal and Performance IQs. These laterality-performance relationships contrasted to the normal readers who only produced one significant effect: they were better in WRAT Arithmetic if they were lateralized poorly. For a stronger test of the functional significance of the dichotic scores, step-wise multiple regression analyses were conducted.

Regression Results

This section is limited to describing the dyslexics' results. With the four

Table 4. Correlations by order between the dichotic lambda scores, IQ and the criterion measures for the Dyslexics and Normals

Measures	Group	Directed Left LF	Directed Left RF	Directed Right LF	Directed Right RF
Verbal IQ[a]					
	Dyslexic	0.16	0.14	0.49**	0.25
	Normals	0.05	0.01	−0.03	−0.06
Performance IQ[a]					
	Dyslexic	0.27	0.20	0.36**	0.22
	Normals	−0.07	0.03	0.01	0.11
Word Attack[b]					
	Dyslexic	−0.64**	−0.34*	0.03	0.27
	Normals	0.14	0.25	0.05	0.02
Passage Comprehension[b]					
	Dyslexic	−0.01	−0.24	0.06	−0.05
	Normals	0.01	−0.02	−0.04	0.07
Reading[c]					
	Dyslexic	−0.30*	−0.22	0.02	−0.09
	Normals	0.07	0.12	−0.16	−0.26
Spelling[c]					
	Dyslexic	−0.32*	−0.31*	0.05	−0.03
	Normals	−0.25	−0.18	−0.19	−0.29
Arithmetic[c]					
	Dyslexic	−0.06	−0.13	0.18	0.08
	Normals	−0.26	0.03	−0.35*	−0.48**

* $p < 0.05$.
** $p < 0.01$.
Partial correlations controlling for Age, Verbal IQ, and Performance IQ produced the same results.
LF = left first order and RF = right first order.
[a] Subtests of the Wechsler Intelligence Scale for Children-Revised.
[b] Subtests of the Woodcock Reading Mastery Test-Revised.
[c] Subtests of the Wide Range Achievement Test-Revised.

dichotic lambda scores, two IQ scores, and CA entered as predictors of the Woodcock and WRAT tests, two significant effects were found. As shown in Figure 2, attending to the LE first was a significant predictor of pseudoword decoding on the Woodcock Word Attack Test, $R^2 = 0.42$, and the slope of the regression line was negative, Beta = −0.80. On the other hand, Verbal IQ predicted performance in Woodcock Passage Comprehension, $R^2 = 0.18$, Beta = 0.42. Neither DAD or IQ predicted any other achievement measure. Entering the four dichotic lambda scores, the other IQ score, and CA as predictors of IQ, showed that recall at the LE second was a significant predictor of both Verbal IQ, $R^2 = 0.24$, Beta = 0.49, and Performance IQ, $R^2 = 0.13$, Beta = 0.36.

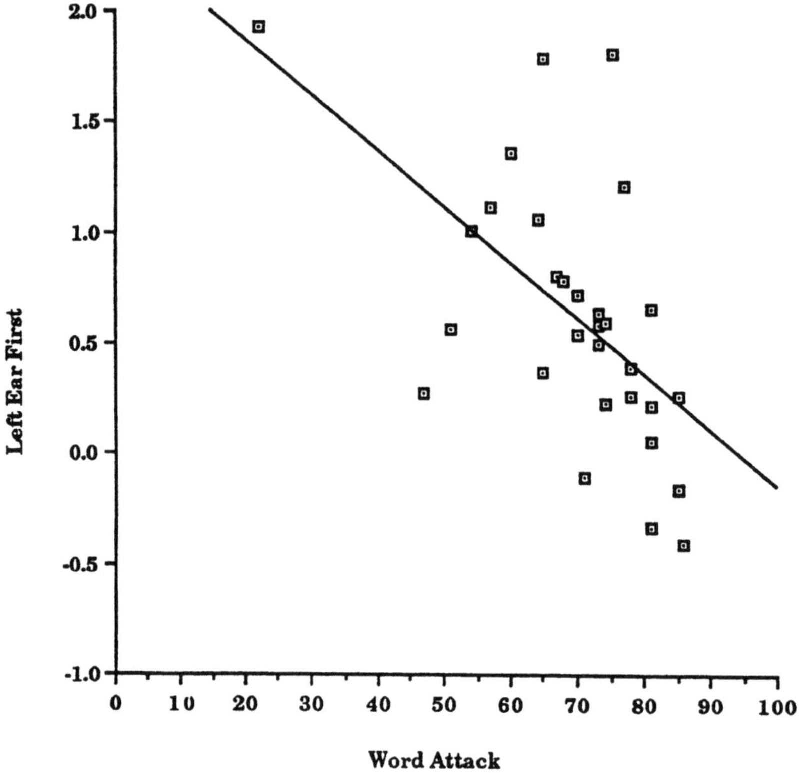

Fig. 2. Scatter-plot of the Regression of Left Ear First Lambda on Word Attack for the Dyslexics.

In summary, the correlational and regression results show: (1) in contrast to younger normal readers, in dyslexics there was no relationship between phonological decoding and reading comprehension but there was a positive relationship between verbal IQ and reading comprehension; (2) dyslexic children's ability to shift from left to right in dichotic listening was related positively to their general intellectual quotients; and (3) a significant predictor of the severity of their phonological word decoding deficit was their facility in attending selectively to the left dichotic channel. Thus those dyslexics who were more weakly lateralized *because they were better in LE recall* were relatively more disabled in pseudoword decoding.

DISCUSSION

When combined with two previous studies addressing the question

(Kershner and Morton, 1990), these results support a modified version of Orton's (1937) claim for a clinically significant relationship between maladaptive cerebral lateralization and dyslexia.

There are, however, substantial changes. Foremost among these is the repeated demonstration, replicated here, that dyslexic children do not differ from normal readers in which hemisphere is lateralized for processing meaningful speech and they do not differ in the degree of left hemisphere linguistic superiority. Approximately 65 percent of the children in both reading groups obtained an REA, which is comparable to other dichotic digit studies with children (Bryden and Allard, 1976). Although the groups were different in age, in view of the impressive evidence that the REA remains invariant throughout childhood (Hiscock, 1988) the age mismatch is unlikely to have influenced this result. It is always possible, of course, that the dichotic test may not be sensitive to dyslexia differences in cerebral asymmetries or that this experiment may have failed to detect group laterality differences because of low statistical power, i.e., sample size and error variance relative to the effect size. However, DAD studies with a range of design characteristics have been consistent in failing to reject the null hypothesis (Obrzut, 1988). Furthermore, alternative approaches to DAD using auditory event-related potentials (Shucard, Cummings and McGee, 1984), regional cerebral blood flow (Hynd, Hynd, Sullivan, and Kingsbury, 1987; Rumsey and Hamburger, 1990), and monaural verbal reaction time (Rastatter, Watson, and Shulman, 1990) have shown that under certain tasks learning disabled subjects, indeed, are more lateralized than normals. Thus the present results add to the increasing volume of converging evidence that dyslexic children are not suffering from incomplete lateralization.

However, consistent with Orton's thinking, dyslexic children who were less lateralized were relatively poorer in pseudoword decoding and, independently, in verbal and performance IQ. But, Orton's conceptualization was premised on stable between-group differences in cerebral asymmetries; no acknowledgement was made of the possibility for qualitatively different fluctuations in lateralized processing in dyslexia as a result of task-specific attentional demands. In the present study, less lateralizaton in the dyslexic children refers to within-group differences in their ability to attend selectively to particular ear-order conditions. Hence, the significance of lateralization to dyslexia appears to be in the dynamic interaction of hemispheric attentional/arousal processes with cerebral asymmetries. This theoretical distinction between lateralized attention and lateralization for processing cognitive content is a second major change from Orton's original model and it, too, is consistent with more recent interpretations of research (Kershner, 1988; Obrzut, 1988; Roeltgen and Roeltgen, 1990).

The most significant outcome of the present study is that 42 percent of the dyslexics' ability to decode pseudowords was accounted for by their ease in recalling from the LE. Important qualifications of this effect are: (1) that it was independent of IQ; and (2) that higher LE scores were related to more severe phonological deficits. This outcome has ramifications for the neuropsychology of dyslexia and for DAD research. Pseudoword decoding is one of the best measures of phonological sensitivity to real words and has been linked etiologically to the disorder (Vellutino et al., 1990). Such findings suggest that LE digit recall, which was unrelated to IQ, may be a valid measure of the hemispheric processes that underlie dyslexia, which by definition is also independent of IQ (Stanovich, 1988). Attending left, again independently of IQ, was also related to the dyslexics' word recognition and spelling; but not to reading comprehension or arithmetic which were IQ-dependent. Furthermore, the power to predict significant variance in pseudoword decoding is noteworthy in the context of other studies. Vellutino (1990), for instance, with a sample of 73 reading disabled children in the same age range, was able to predict 46 percent of the variance in pseudoword decoding; but the final regression involved four obviously more closely related independent variables: phoneme location; phonological memory; WISC-R similarities; and phoneme articulation.

These findings provide fairly clear support for the main hypothesis of the study. It is suggested that spatial attentional demands in dyslexia may promote an exuberance in right hemisphere activation which, in turn, interferes specifically with the development of phonological skills by the left hemisphere. Further evidence consistent with this conclusion comes from an event-related potential (ERP) study comparing dyslexics with normals and with attention-deficit disordered children in a visual-spatial orienting task. Harter, Anllo-Vento, and Wood (1989), in response to contralateral stimuli found an IQ-independent enhancement of N1 in dyslexics over the occipital-central areas, particularly over the right hemisphere, and an IQ-related depression of P3, a measure of post-orienting selection, over the left occipital hemisphere.

Specific modularized neuronal systems are implicated by these results. Moreover, they suggest a neuropsychological link between the underlying neuroanatomical substrates of dyslexia (Galaburda, Rosen, and Sherman, 1990; Geshwind and Galaburda, 1985; Hynd, Semrud-Clikeman, Loreys, Novey, and Eliopulos, in press) and the core deficit in word recognition that marks the disorder clinically (Vellutino et al., 1990). The results suggest a two-factor theory of dyslexia. For instance, work by Galaburda and his colleagues indicates that the brains of dyslexics deviate from the normal pattern of asymmetry of the planum temporale (left larger than right). The more symmetrical dyslexic brains were found to possess larger right hemispheres and were suspected to contain a greater number of callosal terminations (Galaburda et al., 1990). However, the 30 percent incidence of symmetrical plana in normal brains suggests that symmetry may be a necessary but not sufficient, predisposing condition for dyslexia. Indeed, a magnetic resonance imaging study has reported symmetrical plana in all of the disabled children studied who had "pure" phonological deficits (Larsen, Hoien, Lundberg, and Odegaard, 1990). It seems reasonable to hypothesize that plana symmetry may be associated with enhanced right hemisphere spatial attention, but that this, by itself, may not produce dyslexia. A second anatomical feature that has been found in postmortem examinations of dyslexic brains is a large number of neuronal irregularities and these appear primarily in left perisylvian cortex (Kaufman and Galaburda, 1989). Thus, left hemisphere cortical microdysgenesis may need to co-occur with symmetrical plana to produce the phonological word decoding deficits characteristic of dyslexia. Our results suggest that the neuropsychological mechanism functionally connecting these two independent architectural features of the brain with behavior may be an attentional system localized in the right hemisphere that has the potential to interfere transcallosally with phonological processing localized in the left hemisphere.

A few additional comments are in order. Foremost are the limitations of the study. It is highly likely that age-related differences in cognitive strategies and processes were masked by the absence of group differences in DAD. The children in all likelihood were performing at the same level for somewhat different reasons and the impact of the age differences on the regression results is unknown. Additionally, the normal readers were better in pseudoword decoding compared to the dyslexics, which raises the possibility of a development effect confounding the regression results. Control groups of age-matched and younger average readers who are matched with the dyslexics on pseudoword decoding would help to clarify these points. Also, contrary to prediction, dichotic shifting from left to right in the dyslexics was unrelated to pseudoword decoding. Instead, it was related to verbal and performance IQ. This result shows that forced left attending, without the influence of priming shifts in either direction, is the purest dichotic measure of the dyslexics' deficit. Finally, a strength of the younger, reading level-matched control group is that it gives some assurance that our results are not an artifact of less exposure to print in the dyslexics. While a causal connection between attentional lateralization and dyslexia cannot be claimed, the absence of any such relationship in the younger normal readers makes such a claim plausible.

ACKNOWLEDGMENT

Supported by grants from OISE and the Natural Sciences and Engineering Research Council of Canada to the first author.

We gratefully acknowledge the cooperation of the students, their parents, and the staff of the Metropolitan Separate School Board, Toronto.

We thank Dr. Evelyne Corcos for valuable research assistance throughout the study and we thank Sonia DePasqua for her expertise in typing the manuscript.

NOTE

[1] Based on the fourth in a series of lectureships awarded to outstanding scholars by the New York Academy of Medicine as a memorial to Thomas William Salmon, M.D.

REFERENCES

Andersson, B. and Hugdahl, K. (1987). Effects of sex, age, and forced attention on dichotic listening in children: A longitudinal study. *Development Neuropsychology, 3*, 191—206.

Berninger, V. and Traweek, D. (1990). Educational intervention for neuropsychological subtypes of reading disability. Presented at *XVI International Rodin Remediation Scientific Conference*. Boulder, September, 127pp.

Bryden, M. and Allard, F. (1976). Dichotic listening and the development of linguistic processes. In M. Kinsbourne (Ed.), *Hemispheric asymmetries of function* (pp. 127—160). Cambridge, England: Cambridge U. Press.

Bryden, M. and Sprott, D. (1981). Statistical Determination of Degree of Laterality. *Neuropsychologia, 19*, 571—581.

Bryden, M. (1988). Does laterality make any difference? Thoughts on the relation between cerebral asymmetry and reading. In D. Molfese and S. Segalowitz (Eds.), *Brain lateralization in children* (pp. 509—525). NY: Guilford Press.

Galaburda, A., Rosen, G. and Sherman, G. (1990). Individual variability in cortical organization: Its relationship to brain laterality and implications to function. *Neuropsychologia, 28*, 529—546.

Geffen, G. and Wale, J. (1979). Development of selective listening and hemispheric asymmetry. *Developmental Psychology, 15*, 138—146.

Geschwind, N. and Galaburda, A. (1985). Cerebral lateralization. Biological mechanisms, associations, and pathology: II. A hypothesis and a program for research. *Archives of Neurology, 42*, 521—552.

Gladstone, M. and Best, C. (1985). Developmental dyslexia: The potential role of interhemispheric collaboration in readıng acquisition. In C. Best (Ed.), *Hemıspheric function and collaboration in the child* (pp. 87—118). NY: Academic Press.

Harter, M., Anllo-Vento, L. and Wood, F. (1989). Event-related potentials, spatial orienting, and reading dısabilities. *Psychophysiology, 26*, 404—421.

Hiscock, M. (1988). Behavioral asymmetries in normal children. In D. Molfese and S. Segalowitz (Eds.), *Brain lateralization ın children* (pp. 84—169). NY: Guilford Press.

Hynd, G., Hynd, C., Sullivan, H. and Kingsburg, T. (1987). Regional cerebral blood flow in developmental dyslexia: Activation during reading in a surface and a deep dyslexic. *Journal of Learning Dısabilıties, 20*, 294—300.

Hynd, G., Semrud-Clikeman, M., Lorys, A., Novey, E. and Eliopulos, D. (in press). Brain morphology in developmental dyslexia and attention deficit disorder/hyperactivity. *Archives of Neurology.*

Jastak, J. and Wilkinson, G. (1984). *Wide Range Achievement Test-Revised.* Wilmington, DL: Jastak Associates.

Kaufmann, W. and Galaburda, A. (1989) Cerebrocortical microdysgenesis in neurologically normal subjects. *Neurology, 39,* 238—244.

Kershner, J. and Chyczij, M. (in preparation). Lateralized attention in 6—9 year olds and relationships to cognitive development.

Kershner, J. and Morton, L. (1990). Directed attention dichotic listening in reading disabled children: A test of four models of maladaptive lateralization. *Neuropsychologia, 28* 181—198.

Kershner, J. (1988). Dual processing models of learning disability. In D. Molfese and S. Segalowitz (Eds.), *Brain lateralization in children* (pp. 527—546). NY: Guilford Press.

Kinsbourne, M. (1970). The cerebral basis of lateral asymmetries in attention. *Acta Psychologia, 33,* 192—201.

Larsen, J., Hoien, T., Lundberg, I. and Odegaard, H. (1990). MRI evaluation of the size and symmetry of the planum temporale in adolescents with developmental dyslexia. *Brain and Language, 39,* 289—301.

Liberman, I. and Shankweiler, D. (1979). Speech, the alphabet and teaching to read. *In* L. Resnick and P. Weaver (Eds.), *Theory and practice of early reading, Volume II* (pp. 109—132). Hillsdale, NJ: Lawrence Erlbaum.

Mamen, M., Ferguson, B., and Backman, J. (1986). No difference represents a significant finding: The logic of the reading level design. A response to Bryant and Goswami. *Psychological Bulletin, 100,* 104—106.

Obrzut, J. (1988). Deficient lateralization in learning disabled children. In D. Molfese and S. Segalowitz (Eds.), *Brain lateralization in children* (pp. 567—589). NY: Guilford Press.

Orton, S. (1937). *Reading, writing and speech problems in children.* NY: Norton.

Rastatter, M., Watson, M. and Shulman, B. (1990). Neurolinguistic organization in learning disabled children and adoleslcents: Some evidence from monaural, verbal reaction time. *Learning Disabilities Research, 5,* 79—87.

Reuter-Lorenz, P. and Fendrich, R. (1990). Orienting attention across the vertical meridian: Evidence from callosotomy patients. *Journal of Cognitive Neuroscience, 2,* 232—238.

Roeltgen, M. and Roeltgen, D. (1990). Asymmetric lateralized attention in childlren. *Developmental Neuropsychology, 6,* 25—37.

Rumsey, J. and Hamburger, S. (1990). Neuropsychological findings in men with severe developmental dyslexia. *Journal of Clinical and Experimental Neuropsychology, 12,* 70.

Shucard, D., Cummings, K. and McGee, M. (1984). Event-related potentials differentiate normal and disabled readers. *Brain and Language, 21,* 318—334.

Stanovich, K. (1988). Explaining the difference between the dyslexic and the garden-variety poor reader: The phonological-core variable-difference model. *Journal of Learning Disabilities, 21,* 590—604.

Vellutino, F. (1990). Components of variance in reading ability. Implications for the question of subtypes. Presented at *XVI International Rodin Remediation Scientific Conference.* Boulder, September, 17 pp.

Vellutino, F., Scanlon, D. and Tanzman, M. (1990). Differential sensitivity to the meaning and structural attributes of printed words in poor and normal readers. *Learning and Individual Difference, 2,* 19—43.

Vellutino, F. (1979). *Dyslexia: Theory and research.* Cambridge: MIT Press.

Wechsler, D. (1974). *Manual for the Wechsler Intelligence Scale for Children-Revised.* NY: Psychological Corp.

Woodcock, R. (1987). *Woodcock Reading Mastery Tests-Revised.* Circle Pines, MN: American Guidance Service.

Vocabulary Acquisition and Reading Ability

LINDA AGUIAR[1] and SUSAN BRADY[2]

[1] *University of Rhode Island, Kingston, Rhode Island;* [2] *University of Rhode Island, Kingston, Rhode Island and Haskins Laboratories, New Haven, Connecticut*

ABSTRACT: Lexical acquisition ability for aurally taught words was studied in fourth-grade children. Reading ability, intelligence, and working memory were evaluated as predictor factors in vocabulary learning. Reading ability was found to predict facility at learning the novel phonological sequences, while intelligence was the only factor which accounted for performance level for the semantic content of the words. The working memory measure, digit span, failed to make a significant contribution to either the phonological or semantic outcome measures. Examination of two subgroups of skilled and less-skilled readers indicated that less-skilled readers had more difficulty acquiring the phonological information for new words. No between-group differences were found in long-term retention or in the ability to provide definitions for the newly learned words. The findings suggest that the vocabulary deficits of less-skilled readers stem, at least in part, from difficulty establishing accurate phonological representations for new words.

KEYWORDS: lexical acquisition, phonological deficits, reading disability, vocabulary

Vocabulary differences between groups of reading disabled children and their normally achieved peers are often reported (e.g., Kail and Leonard, 1986; Vellutino and Scanlon, 1987). In comparing groups that had been used for research studies, Vellutino and Scanlon noted that the reading disabled groups consistently scored lower than the non-disabled groups on measures of both productive and receptive vocabulary. These differences remained even when the groups were matched on nonverbal IQ performance.

Vocabulary deficits in less-skilled readers are no doubt reciprocally related to reading ability. Poor readers generally read less and therefore could be hampered in vocabulary development by less exposure to print (Cunningham and Stanovich, in press; Hayes, 1988; Nagy and Anderson, 1984; Pratt and Brady, 1988; Stanovich, 1986). In addition, children with impoverished vocabularies find it more difficult to comprehend and recall text (Beck, Perfetti, and McKeown, 1982), which may in turn make it more difficult to incorporate words encountered in text into the mental lexicon (Daneman and Green, 1986; Jenkins, Stein, and Wysocki, 1984; though see Nagy, Anderson, and Herman, 1987, for contrary evidence).

Yet vocabulary deficits in disabled readers are not likely to be merely the consequence of less reading experience. Differences in vocabulary knowledge have been observed in very young poor readers (Gathercole,

Reading and Writing: An Interdisciplinary Journal 3: 413–425, 1991.
© 1991 *Kluwer Academic Publishers.*

Willis, and Baddeley, submitted), raising questions about other factors in vocabulary acquisition. Learning a new word requires accurate perception, storage, and retrieval of the word. Since poor readers have been found to have phonological deficits in each of these areas of processing (for reviews, see Brady, 1991; Liberman and Shankweiler, 1989; and Stanovich, 1985), one might expect them to demonstrate difficulties in vocabulary acquisition, even when new words are encountered outside of text, or aurally. Preliminary evidence confirmed this expectation: Nelson and Warrington (1980) found that a group of dyslexic children produced more errors than a control group on a task of aural vocabulary learning.

Further support for the role of underlying phonological processes in vocabulary learning has come from studies of populations other than the reading disabled. For example, Baddeley, Papagno, and Vallar (1988) reported on the case of an adult patient with a severe deficit in phonological memory who was also deficient on a task of learning nonsense words. Similarly, an association between phonological memory performance and vocabulary acquisition has been reported for prereaders (Gathercole and Baddeley, 1989). Four-year-old children with poor verbal memory scores had smaller receptive vocabularies than those children with better memory performance. A year later, the children who initially had poor phonological recall scores showed lower vocabulary gains, even when the analysis statistically controlled for original vocabulary knowledge. Two studies with adults likewise report a significant correlation between performance on a verbal memory task and achieved vocabulary (Baddeley, Logie, Nimmo-Smith, and Brereton, 1985; Daneman and Green, 1986).

In the present study we wanted to develop a vocabulary learning task in order to confirm whether poor readers have more difficulty acquiring auditorily presented words and to begin investigating underlying phonological factors that may play a role. For this purpose, a game was created in which children help a robot learn words needed for a journey to a distant planet. Fourth-grade children with a broad range of reading skills were taught six new words in the context of this game. We hypothesized that the phonological deficits characteristic of less-skilled readers would impair acquisition of new phonological sequences, but would not impede learning the semantic content. Vocabulary acquisition was scored in terms of phonological errors during training, trials to criterion for correctly producing the words, ability to define the words, and recall and recognition of the new words. Reading ability, intelligence, and working memory were evaluated as predictor factors in vocabulary learning. Performance was assessed for the entire group of subjects and for two sub-groups of skilled and less-skilled readers.

METHOD

Subjects

Subjects were 68 fourth-grade students from a school system in northeastern Rhode Island. The subjects ranged in age from 9 years, 5 months to 10 years, 6 months to limit inclusion to those who had started school at the ages recommended by the school department. Subjects were required to have English as their first language, and to have no known speech or auditory handicaps. In addition, children selected for inclusion scored within the average range on a nonverbal task (the Block Design Subtest of the Wechsler Intelligence Scale of Children-Revised (WISC-R)) (Wechsler, 1974) and were within normal limits on at least one of two verbal measures administered [the Peabody Picture Vocabulary Test-Revised (PPVT-R) (Dunn and Dunn, 1981) and the vocabulary subtest of the WISC-R]. Nine potential subjects were dropped from the final analysis because of failure to meet one or more of the above criteria. One additional subject was dropped because of incomplete data, and two more were eliminated because they failed to reach criterion on the vocabulary learning task within the period allowed in the experiment (see below). The characteristics of the remaining 56 subjects are summarized in Table 1.

Reading groups were formed by using two subtest scores, Word Identification (ID) and Word Attack (ATTACK) from the Woodcock

Table 1. Means for total group of subjects and for two subgroups of skilled and less-skilled readers

	Total group		Skilled readers		Less-skilled readers	
	n = 56		n = 12		n = 10	
	M	(SD)	M	(SD)	M	(SD)
Age	9.8	(0.1)	9.8	(0.3)	9.8	(0.3)
Word ATTACK	6.8	(3.4)	11.3	(2.3)	3.5	(1.1)
Word ID	5.9	(1.7)	8.4	(1.4)	4.1	(0.6)
ESTIQ	106.7	(10.0)	115.5	(12.0)	99.5	(11.9)
PPVT-R	109.2	(13.4)	115.1	(16.0)	103.1	(6.7)
DIGIT	9.6	(2.6)	10.9	(2.4)	8.6	(2.6)
TRIALS	10.6	(3.5)	8.7	(0.8)	11.4	(3.5)
ERRORS	10.2	(6.2)	6.1	(1.6)	10.9	(4.4)
RECALL	1.3	(1.1)	1.8	(1.2)	1.1	(1.0)
RECOG-ST	5.3	(1.1)	5.8	(0.4)	4.6	(1.2)
RECOG-LT	5.4	(0.9)	5.5	(0.6)	5.5	(0.6)
DEFIN	10.0	(5.6)	13.0	(4.2)	8.8	(4.8)

Reading Mastery Test (Woodcock, 1973). Children were ranked according to their scores on these subtests. If a child ranked in the top third of the scores on both subtests, the child was included in the skilled reader group. If a child ranked in the bottom third on both reading measures, the child was included in the less-skilled reading group. Using this method, twelve children fell into the skilled reader group and ten were in the less-skilled reader group. (See Table 1 for descriptive characteristics of the two reading groups.)

Procedure

Each child was tested in three sessions. During the first session, IQ, reading, and working memory measures were administered. In the second session, the children were taught six new words and were then tested for recall and recognition of the trained words. Recognition of the words was again assessed at a third session, conducted at an interval of between one and three weeks from the date of the second session. (The time intervals between sessions two and three were evenly distributed between the reading groups.)

Materials

Predictor measures. All subjects were assessed for reading ability, IQ, and working memory to enable us to examine how strongly each factor related to lexical acquisition ability. As noted above, the Word Identification and Word Attack subtests of the Woodcock Reading Mastery test were utilized to evaluate reading ability. IQ was assessed in two ways. First, the Peabody Picture Vocabulary Test-Revised was administered. Second, the Short form of the WISC-R was given. This includes the Block Design Subtest and the Vocabulary Subtest. An estimated IQ (ESTIQ) was calculated for each subject based on a combination of the two subtest scores as suggested by Sattler (1982). Verbal working memory was assessed with the Digit Span Subtest of the WISC-R (DIGIT).

Experimental Procedure and Materials

Vocabulary Training. Six nonsense words were created for use in this study. Each word was paired with a definition having multiple semantic attributes (see Table 2 for a list of the words and definitions). No one-word English equivalent exists for any of the experimental words. Pictures for each word were painted on 11" × 14" white poster boards.

Each subject was told that they were going to play a game with a robot named Robie. They were told, "Robie is going on an imaginary journey to an imaginery planet. This beautiful planet is golden and has four purple

Table 2. Novel words and definitions

Biffet	— a strange, bald, friendly animal
Corbealyon	— a small, hairy, angry bird
Groshumble	— soft, bouncy, bubble-shaped rain
Pogamer	— a dark and noisy island floating above the ocean
Rimple	— irregularly-shaped, white berries; can be used for robot fuel
Taysum	— a smart, helpful, talking fish

moons. Robie will bring back information about the planet to scientists on Earth. To do this he must enter the information into his memory banks, but sometimes Robie forgets the words he is supposed to remember. Your part in the game is to tell Robie what he needs to remember. These are pictures of what Robie will see on the planet. After you learn the words for them, you will be able to help Robie."

The words were taught to the child in blocks of three. Each of the three words was pronounced and defined while the picture was being shown. The child repeated the word (with correction, if necessary). At the end of the block of three words, the experimenter displayed the pictures for those items and asked the child to name them. (If errors were made, the child was corrected after all three had been shown.) The same group of three words was then presented in another trial block. The order of the words within each block varied. A word was counted as learned if it was correctly produced by the child on two successive blocks of trials. Each group of words was presented at least four times regardless of whether or not the criterion of two successful recalls for all three words had been met. A maximum of ten trials was selected as a cut-off. Children who did not reach the criterion of two consecutive successful trials for each word were not considered for inclusion in the study. (Two children, one skilled reader and one less-skilled reader, were eliminated from the experiment on this basis.) After the first group of three words was learned, the second group was taught using the same procedure.

Performance during the training period was scored for the number of times a block of three words was presented until all three words were learned (TRIALS; possible scores, 4—20). In addition, the number of errors made during vocabulary training was calculated (ERRORS; possible scores, 0—48). The following were classified as errors: 1) a phonologically incorrect form of the target; 2) a phonologically correct or incorrect form of another experimental word; or 3) any other word or a failure to respond.

Assessing Knowledge of Definitions. Immediately following the training, the examiner said the words and asked the child to supply the definitions. If the child did not correctly pair the words and the definitions during testing, the examiner paired the definition components given by the child with the appropriate target. This corrective feedback was given only after all six definitions had been tested. Scores were obtained by counting the number of components of each definition which the child supplied. The total definition score (DEFIN; possible scores, 0—24) was calculated by tallying the semantic characteristics provided for all six words.

Recall and Recognition. Following the training phase, children were introduced to the robot (a small, remote-controlled robot with a tape deck). Short-term recall was then assessed in a game. The robot described an encounter with an object on the planet in terms which closely matched the learned definitions. The child was then asked to provide the correct target word for each given definition. (Example: Robot, "It is almost time for me to go now. I think my fuel is getting low. I have been told that robot fuel grows on this planet. I see some bushes with white berries of many different shapes. Is this robot fuel? What is it called?") All six words were used in the game. The number of words correctly recalled when presented with the definitions were totalled for a recall score (RECALL; possible scores, 0—6).

Following the game, a recognition task was administered. The children were given a booklet containing the pictures of several items on each page. The child was asked by the experimenter to mark a particular target on each page. The number of targets correctly chosen were tallied for a recognition score (RECOG-ST; possible scores: 0—6).

Long-term recognition. A repeat of the booklet task was done at an interval of between one and three weeks from the initial presentation. In this session the robot said the words. A long-term recognition score was tallied for the number of targets correctly chosen (RECOG-LT; possible scores: 0—6.) Plans to also repeat the recall task during this session were abandoned because performance on the initial recall task had been low for all subjects.

RESULTS

The purpose of this study was to examine factors related to lexical acquisition ability in fourth-grade children. We were particularly interested in the the association between reading level and the ability to learn new words. The results were analyzed for the entire group of subjects and for two subgroups of skilled and less-skilled readers.

Evaluation of the Entire Group of Subjects

Several multiple regressions were performed to assess which factors (reading ability, IQ, digit span) best related to the various aspects of vocabulary learning performance. In selecting the variables to be entered into the multiple regression analyses we were concerned to minimize problems arising from multicolinearity between measures (See Table 3 for a correlation matrix for all measures.) The two IQ estimates (PPVT-R and ESTIQ) had a correlation of 0.53. Since debate continues as to how to assess IQ in poor readers (e.g., using verbal measures, including a mix of verbal and nonverbal tests, or using nonverbal techniques), two complete sets of multiple regressions were performed. One set used the PPVT-R as the predictor variable for intelligence, the other used ESTIQ. The results were comparable, and the regressions which used the ESTIQ are reported below.

A second issue concerned the choice of reading measures. A correlation of 0.71 was obtained between the Word Attack and Word Identification measures. Once again, two separate sets of multiple regressions were executed. A virtually identical pattern of results was obtained. Though Word Identification scores accounted for a slightly higher proportion of variance in the outcome measures, the correlation with ESTIQ was somewhat high (0.44) for this form of analysis, so we report the analyses using Word Attack scores.

When factors potentially related to vocabulary learning were assessed (i.e., intelligence (ESTIQ), reading ability (Word Attack), and memory span (DIGIT)), two findings emerged. First, reading ability was found to make the greatest contribution to performance on the phonological measures of word learning. The regression analyses pertaining to how many blocks of trials (TRIALS) were necessary to learn the phonological sequences and to how many errors of production (ERRORS) were made during those blocks both yielded a single measure, Word Attack, accounting for a significant proportion of variance in performance (TRIALS: F $(1,54) = 5.73$, $p = 0.02$, $R^2 = 0.10$); ERRORS: F $(1,54) = 6.18$, $p = 0.02$, $R^2 = 0.10$). Likewise, when regression analyses were computed for the short-term recall and recognition measures, only the reading ability measure (ATTACK) met the stay requirements for the final models (RECALL: F $(1,54) = 8.14$, $p < 0.01$, $R^2 = 0.13$; RECOG-ST: F $(1,54) = 6.83$; $p < 0.01$, $R^2 = 0.11$). In contrast, the intelligence measure was the only factor accounting for a significant proportion of the variance for the semantic outcome measure (DEFIN: F $(1,54) = 21.5$, $p < 0.001$, $R^2 = 0.29$) or for the measure of long-term recognition (RECOG-LT: F $(1,54) = 5.98$, $p < 0.02$, $R^2 = 0.10$). Thus, there is an interesting difference between the factors influencing the acquisition of phonological patterns and the factors relevant to the long-term and semantic aspects of word learning. The working memory measure (DIGIT) failed to make a significant contribution to any of the vocabulary acquisition outcome measures.

Table 3. Intercorrelations among variables in the study (n = 56)

Variable	1	2	3	4	5	6	7	8	9	10
1. Word ID										
2. Word ATTACK	0.71**									
3. ESTIQ	0.44**	0.33*								
4. PPVT-R	0.53**	0.18	0.53**							
5. DIGIT	0.20	0.32*	0.08	−0.03						
6. TRIALS	−0.36**	−0.31*	−0.21	−0.30*	−0.22					
7. ERRORS	−0.35**	−0.32*	−0.22	−0.23	−0.21	−0.88**				
8. RECALL	0.38**	0.36**	0.31*	0.26	−0.06	−0.13	−0.12			
9. RECOG-ST	0.36**	0.27**	0.31*	0.41**	0.11	−0.23	−0.17	0.28*		
10. RECOG-LT	0.14	0.06	0.32**	0.42**	0.14	−0.11	−0.03	0.29*	0.60**	
11. DEFIN	0.29*	0.15	0.53**	0.44**	0.17	−0.18	−0.09	0.14	−0.17	0.52**

* $p < 0.05$
** $p < 0.01$

Comparison of Skilled and Less-Skilled Readers

As described earlier, we also focussed on two subgroups representing more marked differences in reading ability. The skilled and less-skilled readers differed in initial vocabulary scores as measured on both PPVT-R (F (1,21) = 4.62, p = < 0.04) and the ESTIQ (F (1,21) = 4.96, p < 0.04). To control for differences in previous vocabulary knowledge as well as for potential differences in general aptitude, the ESTIQ score was used as a covariate in ANCOVA analyses.

The reading groups did not differ significantly on the ANCOVA comparing their ability to provide the definitions for the newly learned words. On the other hand, the reading groups were found to differ on several of the phonological measures of word learning performance. Nearly significant group differences were obtained on the ANCOVA examining the number of trials required to learn the words (F (1,19) = 4.11, p < 0.056). On the more sensitive measure of number of phonological errors made during training, the poor readers were found to make a significantly greater number of errors (F (1,19) = 6.59, p < 0.02). The retention measures yielded a mixed pattern of results. Accuracy on the short-term recall measure did not differ for reading-groups, perhaps because performance was uniformly low on this task. However, on the short-term recognition measure, good readers were superior at identifying the words' referents (F (1,19) = 4.97, p < 0.02).

A repeated measures ANOVA, for recognition scores of groups over time (short and long term recognition), failed to produce any significant results. Indeed, both the skilled and less-skilled readers had near perfect performance on the long-term task. This ceiling effect on a fairly simple recognition task may be obscuring ongoing difficulties poor readers encounter retaining phonological sequences. A further concern is whether some of the children may have cheated on the long-term recognition measure which, unlike the other tasks, was administered in small groups. Since a small number of cases of cheating were detected by the tester, the results of this measure must be taken tentatively. On the other hand, the significant correlation between the RECOG-LT measure and the ESTIQ measure for the entire group of subjects suggests that other cognitive or linguistic factors may be more critical for long-term retention.

DISCUSSION

The present study suggests that reading skill is linked with the ability to establish and maintain accurate phonological representations when words are first being learned. Performance on the measures tapping phonological components of word learning, such as the number of errors made producing the phonological sequences during training, was found to be more strongly associated with reading ability than with an estimate of general intelligence. Differences between subgroups of skilled and less-skilled readers were apparent on the phonological measures, even when intelligence, including prior vocabulary knowledge, was statistically controlled. In contrast, there was a lack of correspondence between reading skill and ability to retain the conceptual or semantic information for the new words.

These results, which must be considered preliminary, have several interesting implications. First, it is noteworthy that the occurrence of phonological deficits previously documented for poor readers has been extended to include vocabulary acquisition for words introduced aurally. One consequence is that the gap between reading groups in vocabulary knowledge may be expected to widen over time, not only because of lack of exposure or of so-called "Matthew effects" (where reading experience develops other reading-related cognitive abilities), but also because of more basic linquistic deficits that impede vocabulary learning. Unfortunately, the present study did not allow a careful evaluation of long-term retention of words. In a follow-up study, it would be desirable to modify the procedure to permit a long-term recall task which could provide information about the phonological accuracy of words in the lexicon. In an earlier experiment poor readers were found to have inaccurate phonological descriptions for lexical items (Katz, 1986). Long-term follow-up of trained words could help clarify whether observations such as those by Katz stemmed from poor readers' problems learning the correct pattern initially or from difficulty retaining the pattern once it has been acquired.

A second point is that the cognitive difficulties of poor readers do not appear to arise from the semantic or conceptual components of processing. In the present study, performance recalling the semantic attributes of the word was not strongly tied to reading ability. Similarly, Vellutino, Scanlon, and Tanzman (1990) found poor readers to be as sensitive as better readers to the semantic attributes of printed words. Nonetheless, deficits in vocabulary knowledge can be expected to impede both listening and reading comprehension (Beck et al., 1982).

Third, the current findings have implications for instruction. If teachers assume the learning difficulties of poor readers are specific to reading tasks, they may have unrealistic expectations for other tasks or may fail to make necessary modifications in instructional methods. For example, reading disabled children would appear to require more frequent exposure for mastery of words introduced orally. Likewise, the present study adds to the concerns about how to assess the intellectual abilities of poor readers and about the use of IQ scores in allocating services (Stanovich, in press). The difficulty acquiring new lexical items, and the correspondingly lower vocabulary and verbal IQ scores, may cause some children to fail to meet the criteria of 'adequate intelligence' required to qualify for the dyslexia label (and hence for remedial services). One might argue that these children have an even greater need for extra instruction, and may particularly need the benefits to vocabulary growth and comprehension gained from reading experience (e.g., Hayes, 1988; Stanovich and West, 1989).

The findings reported in this study conform with the considerable evidence for phonological deficits in poor readers, yet the results need to be replicated and extended. The vocabulary learning task used might be altered to provide a better metric of word learning performance. The proporation of variance accounted for in the present study was noteworthy, but low (10%—29%). Perhaps if the total number of words acquired were increased, but if fewer were taught in a single session, sources of variability (such as attention, fatigue, etc.) would diminish.

Related to this, it will be important to further investigate the role of underlying phonological processes in vocabulary learning. In order to learn a newly encountered word, a phonological representation must be created in working memory. In the present study, digit span was used as an estimate of working memory, and this variable was not a good predictor of word learning. Yet, Turner and Engle (1989) note that reading group differences on this task are inconsistent. They suggest using a more complicated measure which involves a background task, to avoid the use of rehearsal and grouping strategies. Alternatively, since vocabulary learning in young children has been strongly linked with the ability to repeat pseudowords (Gathercole and Baddeley, 1989), it would also be worthwhile to use this sort of task when exploring working memory factors associated with poor readers' difficulties acquiring new words.

If the acquired word is to be retained for a longer duration, it is of course necessary to retain the phonological and semantic information in the lexicon. While the phonological representation in working memory will have consequences for the nature of this representation in the lexicon, it is also possible that difficulties in acquiring new vocabulary items may stem from processes entailed in storage or retrieval from the lexical system. Poor readers tend to be slower on tasks requiring the rapid naming of visual stimuli such as colors, numbers, letters, or pictured objects (for reviews see: Stanovich, 1985; Wagner and Torgesen, 1987). They also have been reported to make more errors in retrieving phonologically complex labels (i.e., words such as thermometer or stethoscope (Catts, 1986)). These findings suggest it would be worthwhile to explore what effect differences in naming facility have on vocabulary learning. Likewise, the link between working memory and lexical processes warrants scrutiny. Daneman and Green (1986) found that subjects with poorer memory scores were also slower on a lexical retrieval task.

In closing, poor readers are often found to have smaller vocabularies than their better-reading peers. In the study reported here, it was demonstrated that the ability to establish accurate phonological representations for new words is associated with reading skill, but the ability to learn the semantic attributes of words is not. This intriguing outcome suggests that phonological processes involved in lexical acquisition may play a role in reading-group differences in vocabulary. Since vocabulary knowledge, in turn, is central to comprehension performance, a difficulty acquiring words could have wide-spread repercussions. It will be important to replicate these findings and to explore which aspects of phonological processing are implicated.

ACKNOWLEDGEMENTS

We wish to thank Judith Cicero, Janice Ruggeri, and Linda Stoler for their dedicated help collecting data and scoring protocols, and Janet Kulberg and Jerry Cohen for their generous methodological advice. In addition, we thank the principals, teachers, and staff in the Tiverton Public School System who cooperated with us on this project. Lastly, we want to express our gratitude to the children for their diligent and cheerful participation, and to the parents for allowing their children to be in this study.

This article is based on the Master's thesis of the first author. The research and preparation of the manuscript were supported by a grant to Haskins Laboratories (HD-01994) from the National Institute of Child Health and Human Development. Requests for reprints should be directed to Susan Brady, Haskins Laboratories, 270 Crown Street, New Haven, CT 06510.

REFERENCES

Baddeley, A., Papagno, C. and Vallar, G. (1988). When long-term learning depends on short-term storage. *Journal of Memory and Language, 27,* 586—595.

Baddeley, A., Logie, R., Nimmo-Smith, I. and Brereton, A. (1985). Components of fluent reading. *Journal of Memory and Language, 24,* 119—131.

Beck, I., Perfetti, C. and McKeown, M. (1982). The effects of long-term vocabulary instruction on lexical access and reading comprehension. *Journal of Educational Psychology, 74,* 506—521.

Brady, S. (1991). The role of working memory in reading disability. *In* S. Brady and D. Shankweiler (Eds.), *Phonological Processes in Literacy: A Tribute to Isabelle Y. Liberman.* Hillsdale, NJ: Lawrence Erlbaum Associates.

Catts, H. (1986). Speech production/phonological deficits in reading-disordered children. *Journal of Learning Disabilities, 19,* 504—508.

Cunningham, A. and Stanovich, K. (in press). Tracking the unique effects of print exposure in children: Associations with vocabulary, general knowledge, and spelling. *Journal of Educational Psychology.*

Daneman, M. and Green, I. (1986). Individual differences in comprehending and producing words in context. *Journal of Memory and Cognition, 25,* 1—18.

Dunn, L. M. and Dunn, L. M. (1981). *Peabody Picture Vocabulary Test-Revised,* Circle Pines, MN: American Guidance Services.

Gathercole, S. E. and Baddeley, A. D. (1989). Evaluation of the role of phonological STM in the development of vocabulary in children: a longitudinal study. *Journal of Memory and Language, 28,* 200—213.

Gathercole, S. E., Willis, C., and Baddeley, A. (submitted). Differentiating phonological memory and awareness of rhyme: Reading and vocabulary development in children.

Hayes, D. P. (1988). Speaking and writing: Distinct patterns of word choice. *Journal of Memory and Language, 27,* 572—585.

Jenkins, J., Stein, M. and Wysocki, K. (1984). Learning vocabulary through reading. *American Educational Research Journal, 21,* 767—787.

Katz, R. (1986). Phonological deficiencies in children with reading disability: Evidence from an object-naming task. *Cognition, 22,* 225—257.

Kail, R. and Leonard L. (1986). Word-finding abilities in language impaired children. *ASHA Monographs, 25,* Rockland, MD: American Speech-Hearing-Language Association.

Liberman, I. Y. and Shankweiler, D. P. (1989). Phonology and the beginning reader: A tutorial. *In* L. Rieben et C. A. Perfetti (Eds.), *L'Apprenti lecteur — Apports experimentaux et implications.* Pedagogiques, Neuchatel: Delachaux et Niestle.

Nagy, W. E. and Anderson, R. C. (1984). How many words are there in printed school English? *Reading Research Quarterly, 23,* 304—330.

Nagy, W. E., Anderson, R. C. and Herman, P. (1987). Learning word meaning from context during normal reading. *American Educational Research Journal, 24,* 237—270.

Nelson, H. E. and Warrington, E. K. (1980). An investigation of memory functions in dyslexic children. *British Journal of Psychology, 71,* 487—503.

Pratt, A. and Brady, S. (1988). Relation of phonological awareness and reading ability in children and adults. *Journal of Educational Psychology, 80,* 319—323.

Sattler, J. (1982). *Assessment of Children's Intelligence and Special Abilities.* Boston, MA: Allyn and Bacon.

Stanovich, K. E. (in press). Discrepancy definitions of reading disability: Has intelligence led us astray? *Reading Research Quarterly.*

Stanovich, K. (1985). Explaining the vairance in reading ability in terms of psychological processes: What have we learned? *Annals of Dyslexia, 35,* 67—96.

Stanovich, K. E. (1986). Matthew effects in reading: Some consequences of individual differences in the acquisition of literacy. *Reading Research Quarterly, 21,* 360—407.

Stanovich, K. E. and West, A. (1989). Exposure to print and orthographic processing. *Reading Research Quarterly, 24,* 402—433.

Turner, M. and Engle, R. (1989). Is working memory capacity task dependent? *Journal of Memory and Language, 28,* 127—154.

Vellutino, F. R. and Scanlon, D. M. (1987). Linguistic coding and reading ability. *In* S. Rosenberg (Ed.), *Advances in Psycholinguistics,* (pp. 1—69). New York: Cambridge University Press.

Vellutino, F. R., Scanlon, D. M. and Tanzman, M. (1990). Differential sensitivity to the meaning and structural attributes of printed words in poor and normal readers. *Learning and Individual Differences, 2,* 19—43.

Wagner, R. and Torgesen, J. (1987). The nature of phonological processing and its causal role in the acquisition of reading skills. *Psychological Bulletin, 101,* 192—212.

Wechsler, D. (1974). *Wechsler Intelligence Scale of Children — Revised.* San Antonio, TX: Psychological Corporation.

Woodcock, R. W. (1973). *Woodcock Reading Mastery Tests.* Circle Pines, MN: American Guidance Service.

Discussion

Observations from the Sidelines

A. M. LIBERMAN
Haskins Laborataories, 270 Crown Street, New Haven, CT. 06511

Isabelle Liberman had long believed that if she and her colleagues were to understand dyslexia or, more generally, reading, they had first to deal with the characteristic of language that is most directly relevant: the vast difference in naturalness (hence, difficulty) between its spoken and written forms (Liberman, 1971; Shankweiler and Liberman, 1972; Liberman, I. Y., Shankweiler, and Liberman, A. M., 1989). In a state of nature, everybody speaks, nobody reads. Thus, alexia is the biologically normal condition; what we call dyslexia is simply the inability to rise above it. It therefore seemed to Isabelle the merest common sense to suppose that knowing why reading is relatively difficult for all would likely reveal why it is inordinately difficult for some.

The obvious key to the difference in naturalness between the spoken and written forms of language is in the fact that speech is a species-typical product of biological evolution, while writing systems are artifacts. The less obvious corollary is to be found in the strikingly different ways by which systems with such disparate courses of development meet a requirement that is imposed on all forms of communication, whether evolved or invented. This requirement, which goes to the heart of questions about the genetic and neurological bases of communication, is what Mattingly and I have called 'parity': sender and receiver must be bound by a common understanding that only certain signals, or, more properly, their perceptual representations, have communicative significance; otherwise, communication cannot occur (Mattingly and Liberman, 1988; Liberman and Mattingly, 1989). Given that speech was a result of evolution, not invention, we know that parity cannot have been established by convention. It had, rather, to be built into the underlying biology, and that was accomplished by the development of a specialization for speech, a biologically coherent device specifically adapted to recover the linguistically relevant articulatory gestures of the speaker, and so to produce percepts that are, *ab initio*, of a distinctly phonetic cast. Indeed, speech percepts cannot be auditory in the ordinary sense, for if they were, then only a deliberate cognitive process could have marked them for linguistic significance, and so attached them to language. In that case, our ancestors would have had to agree to call certain otherwise undistinguished auditory representations by phonetic names, and then pledge to use them exclusively for linguistic purposes. But speech percepts did not have to be

Reading and Writing: An Interdisciplinary Journal 3: 429—433, 1991.
© 1991 *Kluwer Academic Publishers.*

named; as Studdert-Kennedy aptly put it, they 'name themselves' (Studdert-Kennedy, 1976). Unlike the ordinary primitives of pitch, loudness, and timbre — primitives that form a countless variety of identifiable percepts — those of the phonetic modality are used only for language; having evolved for a specifically linguistic purpose, they are simply no good for anything else. This is to say that speech percepts are specifically and exclusively phonetic as they are immediately represented to cognition by the speech specialization. No cognitive translation from auditory primitives is necessary. Accordingly, the phonetic representations evoked by the sounds of speech are, by their very nature, integral parts of language; they are not merely vehicles for conveying it. Speech puts the listener immediately into the language system (Liberman and Mattingly, 1985; Mattingly and Liberman, 1988).

A writing system is a different matter altogether. There, the letters of the alphabet evoke percepts that are unremarkably visual; they are not inherently linguistic, for there is no specialization to make them so. Indeed, the probability that there is a specialization for reading is exactly equal to the probability that there is a specialization for playing poker. Therefore, parity can only have been established by convention. Someone had to decide that certain optical shapes, and only those shapes, should be considered to have linguistic significance, which is exactly what it means to say that writing systems are artifacts. In consequence, it is left to the reader to confer linguistic status on nonlinguistic percepts, and this requires of him a cognitive step that the speech perceiver need not take. Of course, a reader might decline to take that step, electing rather to make do with representations that bear no organic relation to language. Thus, at the first stage, the reader might develop a purely visual lexicon. On that strategy, however, he would not only be required to do the same lexical job twice, but, for the purpose of reading, he would be unable to do it the way nature intended. After all, phonological processes evolved as part of the specialization for language just to make it easy for humans to create, acquire, store, and access the tens or hundreds of thousands of words that a lexicon typically comprises.

The price of such a nonlinguistic strategy is seen to be the more steep when one considers that phonological structures are presumably the raw materials on which syntactic processes normally work. Must a reader cobble together a set of cognitive processes that are not specialized for language, and for which he has no natural affinity, just in order to do a syntactic job on representations that remain stubbornly nonphonological? Surely, that would be hard to do; indeed, it might not even be possible.

The seemingly sensible strategy for the reader is to use the optical shapes to access the phonological structures early in the reading process. Once the reader has done that, he has put the hard part of reading behind him, for everything else will be done automatically by language processes that he commands by virtue of his humanity. But connecting the optical characters to the phonology is not so easy as it might seem. At the very least, it requires more than just knowing what is called, in 'phonics' instruction, the 'sounds of the letters'. In fact, learning to attach those sounds to the letters is trivially easy for almost everyone; unfortunately, it is only marginally helpful and may, indeed, be hurtful. As Isabelle pointed out so many times, it avails the reader little to know that the [b], the [a], and the [g] of [bag] are pronounced [buh], [a], and [guh], for that will most likely lead him to [buhaguh], which is the wrong word. What he must know is that a word like [bag] is formed of three phonological units; only then does it make sense to him that it should be spelled with three letters. To see that this is a cognitive achievement of sorts, one need only consider that, while our ancestors had presumably begun to speak about the time they emerged as a distinct species, they had to wait until a few thousand years ago for the discovery by one of their number that every word they spoke had an internal phonological structure. This momentous discovery was readily translated into the alphabetic principle, a triumph of applied biology that was the necessary precondition for the invention of the mode of reading and writing we all use. Unfortunately for the would-be reader, however, the proper use of this invention requires a conscious grasp of the underlying principle, as opposed to a tacit command of the phonological structures it captures, and this conscious grasp does not come as standard equipment on the linguistic faculty we all inherit.

So what stood in the way of the discovery by our ancestors that the words they spoke so effortlessly all had a phonological structure? Why should it have been relatively hard for them, and now for us, to develop what Isabelle and her colleagues have called 'phonological awareness'? The first consideration, of course, is that, as we have already seen, such awareness is not required for speech. In that natural mode, the speaker need only think of the word; the speech specialization spells it for him, automatically selecting and coordinating the gestures that define its phonological units. As for the listener, he need not consciously and effortfully parse the speech signal; again, the speech specialization takes over, recovering the phonological structure that distinguishes the word and forms the basis for all further linguistic work that will be done with it.

Thus, there is nothing in the speaker's experience with speech that requires him to be aware of phonological structure. But there is more to the matter than that, because there *is* something in speech that actually tends to make that awareness more difficult than it would otherwise be. That something is coarticulation, the process that, in all languages, overlaps and merges the gestures that define the phonological elements. This species-specific aspect of the phonetic specialization was critical in the evolution of speech, because it made possible the high rates (reaching 15 or more phonological segments per second) that normal speakers achieve.

It was also critical for speech perception, because, by folding several phonological segments into a single piece of sound, it relaxed the constraint on rate of perception that is set by the temporal resolving power of the ear. But the consequence for the would-be reader is less happy, for he must contend with the fact that, because of coarticulation, the phonological segments do not generally correspond in any straightforward way to the acoustic segments. In a word like [bag], as in most words, the phonological information is so thoroughly overlapped and smeared that there is simply no acoustic criterion by which it can be sorted out and so made perfectly apparent to the consciousness of speaker and listener (Liberman, Cooper, Shankweiler, and Studdert-Kennedy, 1967). Still, the underlying phonological structure *is* available to consciousness, as the existence of skilled readers proves, but only at the cost of a cognitive effort.

Why, then, should the cognitive achievement that phonological awareness represents be more difficult for some than for others. The view favored by Isablle and her colleagues is not that these dyslexics are lacking in cognitive resources, but only that they suffer from a deficiency — presumably a mild one — in the phonological component of their specialization for language, and that this causes some reduction in the clarity or robustness of the phonological representation (Liberman, Shankweiler, and Liberman, 1989). If these representations are weak, then they should be that much less readily available for conscious inspection. But difficulty in achieving phonological awareness should not be the only symptom of a weakness in the phonological system. We should also expect to find constraints on short-term memory for verbal materials (working memory, as it is sometimes called), together with somewhat greater than normal difficulty in perceiving speech in noise, in finding the phonological structures appropriate to naming objects, and, given that production is the other side of the special phonological coin, in executing difficult articulatory maneuvers. As for the genetics and neurology of dyslexia — the subjects of this conference — is it not plausible to suppose that individual differences in a coherent and recently evolved specialization should exist and be heritable?

REFERENCES

Liberman, A. M., Cooper, F. S., Shankweiler, D. P. and Studdert-Kennedy, M. (1967). Perception of the speech code. *Psychology Review, 74,* 431—461.

Liberman, A. M. and Mattingly, I. G. (1985). The motor theory of speech perception revised. *Cognition, 21,* 1—36.

Liberman, A. M. and Mattingly, I. G. (1989). A specialization for speech perception. *Science, 243,* 489—494.

Liberman, I. Y. (1971). Basic research in speech and lateralization of language: Some implications for reading disability. *Bulletin of the Orton Society, 21*, 7–87.
Liberman, I. Y., Shankweiler, D. and Liberman, A. M. (1989). The alphabetic principle and learning to read. In D. Shankweiler and I. Y. Liberman (eds.), *Phonology and reading disability: Solving the reading puzzle.*, IARLD Monograph Series, Ann Arbor, MI: University of Michigan Press.
Mattingly, I. G. and Liberman, A. M. (1988). Specialized perceiving systems for speech and other biologically significant sounds. In G. M. Edelman, W. E. Gall and W. M. Cowan (Eds.), *Functions of the Auditory System.* (pp. 775–793). New York: Wiley.
Shankweiler, D. and Liberman, I. Y. (1972). Misreading: A search for causes. In J. F. Kavanagh and I. G. Mattingly (Eds.), *Language by ear and by eye: The relationships between speech and reading* (pp. 293–317). Cambridge, MA: MIT Press. [Reprinted (1975) in P. H. Mussen, J. S. Conger and J. Kanan (Eds.), *Basic and contemporary issues in development psychology.* New York: Harper & Row.]
Studdert-Kennedy, M. (1976). Speech perception. *In* Lass, N.J. (ed.) *Contemporary Issues in Experimental Phonetics.* New York: Academic Press, pp. 243–293.

Hemispheric Specialisation and Dyslexia

J. F. STEIN
University Laboratory of Physiology, Oxford

In this short paper I would like to attempt to answer the question posed by Professor Alvin Liberman when he asked at this Conference why there is no evidence for a visual linguistic module underlying reading, analogous to the phonological one, which he and his late wife have done so much to show mediates speech (Liberman et al., 1967). In attempting to answer this question I shall raise some further ones which are related.

Probably there are many genes controlling the development of speech and language. But this does not mean that these are the same or the only ones that influence reading. My first question is therefore, why is it so often assumed that the genetics of dyslexia and of language development are necessarily identical? Genetic control is probably exercised over hemispheric specialisation rather than speech, language or reading per se; hence dyslexic children may have deficits related to the functions of both hemispheres. So, my second question is, why do those who look for subgroupings among dyslexics always seem to assume that children must either have phonological or visual perceptual deficits but not both together?

Several presentations at the Conference confirmed that dyslexia is clearly heritable. It is a phonological deficit that most believe causes the trouble. As Al. Liberman puts it, reading is difficult because speaking is so easy. For we speak by means of a continuous series of articulatory gestures which we learn by copying those around us; we do not have to be taught them explicitly. The alphabetic principle is not so easily gained however. In order to learn to read we must learn to segment the continuous stream of sounds which we produce when speaking, not merely into syllables, but into phonemes, in order to be able to associate them with their written equivalents, graphemes. These distinctions are arbitrary and must be taught and learned. Children with impaired phonological development find the identification of the order of sounds difficult; hence it is not surprising that they have great problems learning to read.

Numerous groups around the world have confirmed that may dyslexic children perform poorly in phonological tests, such as reading 'nonwords' (Snowling, 1981), rhyming or alliteration (Bradley and Bryant, 1983). Furthermore Dick Olson and colleagues (1989) and Jim Stevenson (this meeting) have both shown that poor nonword reading performance is heritable; and Olson argues that this accounts for most of the heritability

Reading and Writing: An Interdisciplinary Journal **3**: 435—440, 1991.
© 1991 *Kluwer Academic Publishers.*

of poor reading performance. There is thus clear evidence, with which few disagree, that a major problem which dyslexics face is deficient phonological skill.

Often this problem is associated with a history of difficulties with learning to speak, such as lisping, stuttering, and late development of proper pronounciation. It is therefore reasonable to conclude that dyslexic children suffer a minor impairment of their speech processing system, which Al. Liberman describes as their "encapsulated phonological linguistic module". Since this module is often thought to be confined to the left hemisphere, it is natural to suspect and look for signs of left hemisphere damage in these children.

None of this evidence emphasising dyslexics' phonological impairments excludes the possibility that they may also suffer other impairments however (Snowling, 1987); or indeed that a few might not suffer phonological problems at all. A frequent suggestion has been that dyslexic children may also suffer from visual perceptual problems. Certainly many dyslexics themselves, together with many of their teachers, think there is something wrong with their eyesight. However, just as there is seldom anything wrong with the hearing of those who exhibit phonological problems, so dyslexics normally pass the standard eye tests with flying colors. The current consensus is that there is nothing obviously wrong with their eye movements either (Olson et al., 1983).

More and more evidence is accruing however that higher level visual functions may, after all, be abnormal in dyslexic children. In up to three-quarters their binocular control is unstable (Stein et al., 1988), they have poor stereoacuity (Stein et al., 1987), lowered contrast sensitivity in the mid range of spatial frequencies, impaired temporal resolution (Slaghuis and Lovegrove, 1985) and poor visual direction sense for small targets, such as letters (Riddell et al., 1990). They also show a greater than normal susceptibility to peripheral distractors when attempting to identify small visual targets (Geiger and Lettvin, 1987; Ruddock, 1991). This is known as 'crowding' (Atkinson, 1991).

The high incidence of these problems in dyslexic children suggests that they may often coexist with the phonological problems discussed earlier. Dick Olson found that the heritability of his subjects' poor performance in his phonological task was much greater than that in his orthographic task, which was to identify homophones visually. But if he entered the orthography scores before phonology in his multiple regression model, then the visual modality, orthography, was shown to account for much more of his subjects' variance in heritability of reading ability. This suggests that visuoperceptual factors and phonology may covary very tightly. Indeed Jim Stevenson found that poor homophone recognition was highly heritable, even in children who were merely low normal readers. Moreover Dorothy Bishop pointed out that the ability to place cartoon pictures in the correct order visually to make a coherent story, was a stronger predictor of future language ability in children than any of the phonological tests she employed. It seems therefore that dyslexics may show significant impairments in tests of higher level visual skills, and that these may often coexist with phonological deficits.

How does this relate to A. Liberman's question about a visual linguistic module, its relationship to phonology, and the question of whether there is a gene for reading? Clearly successful reading requires not only phonological, but also visual skills. It seems most unlikely that a cultural achievement which was only invented 2,000 years ago, and only in the last 100 years has been at all widespread, should have a specific gene allocated to it. It is much more likely that reading, like speech, was made possible by the prior evolutionary development of hemispheric specialisation (Stein, 1988). Probably visuospatial functions which require greater precision than can easily be organised by communication between the hemispheres, were evolved first in the right hemisphere (Webster, 1977). Then later the left hemisphere was taken over for the development of accurate vocalisation.

Thus the answer to the question why no visual linguistic module was developed, is that suggested by Al Galaburda. Sound is the natural medium for linguistic communication; and the ear is its sense organ. Hence a phonological linguistic module was developed in the left hemisphere (Liberman et al., 1967). But vision is the medium for visuospatial perception, not language; and the eye is its sensory organ. Specialisation of the right hemisphere therefore evolved for a different kind of task of which the requirements of reading were able to take advantage. The precise binocular control and accurate visual sequencing of small letters required for reading, make especially heavy demands on these right hemisphere functions (Stein, 1991). But this is not a specifically visual linguistic problem; it merely reflects the contribution which the visual system makes to reading. We should not be looking for a separate visual linguistic module therefore, any more than it would be sensible to look to the ear to provide us with visuospatial information.

Nor should we look for a gene for dyslexia; rather we should attempt to clarify the genetic mechanisms that control hemispheric specialisation (Annett, 1985). Herbert Lubs pointed out in this Conference that we need to refine our definition of the dyslexic phenotype, before we can hope to identify the genes responsible. Probably what we need to do is to identify the phenotypic signs of hemispheric specialisation, rather than trying to purify our definition of dyslexia. Then the study of disorders of hemispheric specialisation should help us to clarify the relationship between genetic abnormalities and the signs of altered hemispheric specialisation which may be seen neuroanatomically in CAT, MRI, PET scans (Galaburda, 1988) and brain electrical activity mapping (Duffy,

1986). These should then be interpretable in terms of the altered physiological mechanisms which prevent successful reading. It is now clear that these impaired processing operations will implicate both left and right hemispheres; the leftsided abnormalities giving rise to phonological coding deficiencies; and the rightsided abnormalities giving rise to visuospatial deficiencies, which are no less detrimental to reading progress.

Stein, Eden and Fowler presented evidence at this Symposium that dyslexic children do indeed demonstrate abnormalities of right hemisphere function, particularly involving the right posterior parietal cortex. They showed that two-thirds of dyslexic children have impaired binocular stability which is particularly marked on the left side. They demonstrated that this abnormality causes impaired visuospatial ability. Children who have poor binocular control also show depressed contrast sensitivity in the mid range of spatial frequencies (3 cycles/degree); and they often exhibit mild signs of left sided neglect. They tend to leave out the left hand numbers when drawing a clock and they fail to notice some of the stars on the left in a 'star cancellation' task. In addition to their binocular instability their eye movements are slightly abnormal. Both eyes tend to drift right in the Cover Test, and during smooth pursuit they tend to 'cogwheel'; their eyes lag behind the target and then catch up by means of frequent saccades — saccadic intrusions. They also occasionally make saccades which fall short of the target (hypometric saccades) on the left; and they exhibit a few beats of nystagmus, particularly when the eyes are deviated to the extreme left. These results are sumarized in Stein (1991).

These mild visual abnormalities pointing to abnormal processing in the right posterior parietal cortex should be compared with those of patients with clearly established right posterior parietal lesions (Stein et al., 1989). Such patients have all the foregoing deficiencies, but in a much more extreme form (Heilman and Valenstein, 1985; Stein, 1989; Fowler et al., 1989): their visual acuity is reduced; they have decreased contrast sensitivity over the whole range of spatial frequencies; they exhibit severe neglect of the left side of space, as shown by inability to fill the left side of a clock face, and their tendency to ignore all the stars on the left in the star cancellation task. They are also very inaccurate at localising small dots on their left hand side; and they misaim grossly on the left hand side. Like dyslexic children they have a tendency for both eyes to drift right in the Cover Test. They show much more severe cogwheeling during smooth pursuit than dyslexics, particularly when the eyes are moving out of the affected (left) field; they grossly undershoot targets on the left (hypometric saccades); and they have very poor fusion, absent vergence control and severely reduced stereopsis. By comparison patients with left posterior parietal lesions are, by and large, normal, so far as their visual performance is concerned; although often they have serious aphasic problems (Fowler et al., 1989).

Thus the answer to Al Liberman's question — why is there no visual linguistic module — is that the right hemisphere is specialised not for language, but for visuomotor functions, particularly those involved in fine binocular control and stereopsis. These happen also to be functions required for successful reading. They are not primarily linguistic, unlike the phonological processing operations carried out by the left hemisphere. Hence although there is a specialised phonological linguistic processing module in the left hemisphere, there is no visual linguistic one in the right hemisphere. Instead there is a non-linguistic visuospatial processing module in the right hemisphere. The normal development of both the linguistic and visuospatial modules probably depends upon the genetic mechanisms which control hemispheric specialisation. Thus there are probably no specific genes for language development, still less are there genes for visual linguistic development. If the mechanisms underlying the specialisation of the hemispheres are disordered however the phenotype usually demonstrates signs of both linguistic and visuospatial hemisphere dysfunction.

Thus the answer to the second question with which I began, why is it so often assumed that dyslexics only have phonological or visual problems, but not both, is probably that the two are tightly correlated, because they are consequences of the same genetic process. Since they so often occur together, they are difficult to separate. Tests of phonology are well established and accepted; but what tests of visuomotor control are appropriate for use in dyslexics is still not settled. So the result tends to be that people assume that phonological impairments are the only cause of dyslexia. I hope I have shown in this short paper that this is not necessarily so; and that we should look more closely at the visuomotor functions of the right hemisphere in dyslexic children, because impairments of these may often coexist with disordered phonology.

REFERENCES

Annett, M (1985). *Left and Right, Hand and Brain: The Right Shift Theory.* London: Erlbaum.

Atkinson, J. (1991). Crowding Effects in Young Children and Dyslexics. In Stein, J. F. (Ed.), *Vision and Visual Dyslexia.* New York: Macmillan Press.

Bradley, L. and Bryant, P. E. (1983). Categorizing sounds and learning to read — a causal connection. *Nature, 301,* 419—421.

Duffy, F. H. (1986). 'Topographic Mapping of Brain Electrical Activity (BEAM)'. New York: Butterworths.

Fowler, M. S., Munro, N., Richardson, A. and Stein, J. F. (1989). Vergence control in patients with lesions of the posterior oparietal cortex. *Journal of Physiology, 417,* 92.

Galaburda, A. (1988). The pathogenesis of childhood dyslexics. In F. Plum (Ed.), *Language, Communication and the Brain.* New York: Raven Press.

Geiger, S. and Lettvin, J. Y. (1987). Peripheral vision in persons with dyslexia. *New England Journal of Medicine, 316*, 1238—1243.

Heilman, K. M. and Valenstein, E. (1985). 'Clinical Neuropsychology'. New York: Oxford University Press.

Liberman, A. M., Cooper, F. S., Shankweiler, D. P. and Studdert Kennedy, M. (1967). A motor theory of speech perception. *Psychological Review, 73*, 431—461.

Olson, R. K., Kliegl, R. and Davidson, B. J. (1983). Dyslexic and normal readers' eye movements. *Journal of Experimental Psychology, 9*, 816—825.

Olson, R. K., Wise, B., Conners, F., Rack, J. and Fulker, D. (1989). Specific deficits in component reading and language skills: Genetic and environmental influences. *Journal of Learning Disabilities, 22*, 339—348.

Riddell, P., Fowler, M. S. and Stein, J. F. (1990). Inaccurate visual localisation in dyslexic children. *Perceptual and Motor Skills, 70*, 707—718.

Ruddock, K. H. (1991). Visual Search in Dyslexia. *In*: J. F. Stein (ed.), *Vision and Visual Dyslexia*. New York: Macmillan Press.

Slaghuis, W. and Lovegrove, W. J. (1985). Spatial-frequency mediated visible persistence and specific reading disability. *Brain and Cognition, 4*, 219—240.

Snowling, M. J. (1981). Phonemic defects in developmental dyslexia. *Psychological Research, 43*, 219—234.

Snowling, M. J. (1987). 'Dyslexia — a Cognitive Development Perspective'. Oxford: Blackwell.

Stein, J. F., Riddell, P. M. and Fowler, M. S. (1987). Fine binocular control in dyslexic children. *Eye, 1*, 433—438.

Stein, J. F. (1988). Physiological differences between left and right hemispheres. *In*: F. C. Rose (Ed.), *Aphasia*. London: Whurr Wyke.

Stein, J. F., Riddell, P. and Fowler, M. S. (1988). Disordered vergence eye movement control in dyslexic children. *British Journal of Ophthalmology, 72*, 162—166.

Stein, J. F. (1989). Representation of egocentric space in the posterior parietal cortex. *Quarterly Journal of Experimental Physiology, 14*, 583—606.

Stein, J. F., Riddell, P. M. and Fowler, M. S. (1989). Disordered Right Hemisphere Function in Developmental Dyslexia. In: von Euler (Ed.), 'Brain and Reading'. New York: Macmillan Press.

Stein, J. F. (1991). Visuospatial Sense, Hemispheric Asymmetry and Dyslexia. *In*: J. F. Stein (Ed.), *Vision and visual dyslexia*. New York: Macmillan Press.

Webster, W. (1977). Hemispheric Asymmetry in Cats. *In*: S. Harnad (Ed.), *Lateralization in the nervous system*. New York: Academic Press.

NEUROPSYCHOLOGY AND COGNITION

The purpose of the Neuropsychology and Cognition series is to bring out volumes that promote understanding in topics relating brain and behavior. It is intended for use by both clinicians and research scientists in the fields of neuropsychology, cognitive psychology, psycholinguistics, speech and hearing, as well as education. Examples of topics to be covered in the series would relate to memory, language acquisition and breakdown, reading, attention, developing and aging brain. By addressing the theoretical, empirical, and applied aspects of brain-behavior relationships, this series will try to present the information in the fields of neuropsychology and cognition in a coherent manner.

Series Editor

R. Malatesha Joshi, *Oklahoma State University, U.S.A.*

Publications

1. P.G. Aaron: *Dyslexia and Hyperlexia.* 1989 ISBN 1-55608-079-4
2. R. M. Joshi (ed.): *Written Language Disorders.* 1991 ISBN 0-7923-0902-2
3. A. Caramazza: *Issues in Reading, Writing and Speaking.* A Neuropsychological Perspective. 1991 ISBN 0-7923-0996-0
4. B. F. Pennington (ed.): *Reading Disablities.* Genetic and Neurological Influences. 1991 ISBN 0-7923-1606-1

KLUWER ACADEMIC PUBLISHERS – DORDRECHT / BOSTON / LONDON

MIX
Papier aus verantwortungsvollen Quellen
Paper from responsible sources
FSC® C105338

If you have any concerns about our products,
you can contact us on
ProductSafety@springernature.com

In case Publisher is established outside the EU,
the EU authorized representative is:
Springer Nature Customer Service Center GmbH
Europaplatz 3, 69115 Heidelberg, Germany

Printed by Libri Plureos GmbH
in Hamburg, Germany